SURVIVING:
A COLON CANCER DIARY

Beverly A. Battaglia, Ph.D.

with Amy Law, M.D.

Other books by Beverly Battaglia

CHANGING LANES: COUPLES REDEFINING RETIREMENT

Dr. Battaglia can be reached at Battagltd@aol.com or on her blog site: RetirementConnection.Blogspot.com

ISBN: 13:978-1539315193

10:1539315193

First Printing: October, 2016

ACKNOWLEDGEMENTS

A special thank you to my husband, family and friends, who helped and supported me through my cancer recovery and the later process of writing and producing this book

A special thank you goes to my oncologist, Dr. Amy Law, for her care and support through my recovery process. Dr. Law also encouraged me to share my successful cancer journey by writing a book. She contributed to this book by providing helpful comments and suggestions to assist cancer patients, oncologists, nurses and other personnel. In addition, Dr. Law referred other colon cancer patients, who volunteered to share their stories of recovery.

Another thank you goes to the seven colon cancer patient volunteers, who shared their stories of traversing the unfamiliar maze of cancer procedures to achieve a successful outcome.

I'd like to also acknowledge my editor, Eileen Cinque for her guidance and comments which helped me maneuver my way through the publishing process.

TABLE OF CONTENTS

PREFACE

INTRODUCTION

CHAPTER 1   PRECANCER – EARLY ASSESSMENT

CHAPTER 2   NEXT STEPS – DIAGNOSIS

CHAPTER 3   NEXT STEP – SURGERY

CHAPTER 4   TREATMENT OPTIONS

CHAPTER 5   TREATMENT BEGINS

CHAPTER 6   TREATMENT ISSUES

CHAPTER 7   THE PORT PROBLEM

CHAPTER 8   TREATMENT SESSIONS CONTINUE

CHAPTER 9   POST TREATMENT EXPERIENCE

CHAPTER 10	OTHER SURVIVOR EXPERIENCES
CHAPTER 11	MANAGING CHEMOTHERAPY SIDE EFFECTS
CHAPTER 12	SUPPORT SYSTEMS – FINANCIAL, FAMILY, FRIENDS
CHAPTER 13	FINAL THOUGHTS AND SUMMATION
ADDENDUM	EXPLANATION OF TERMS USED

PREFACE

Changing Lanes II - Cancer Detour

When I wrote *Changing Lanes: Couples Redefining Retirement*, I knew that my retirement road would not always be a straight, easy highway. I had talked with over a hundred retirees who were on the retirement road with me, and they shared their stories of hitting roadblocks, detours and accidents. We all had to search out ways of dealing with the sometimes unexpected events in life. When you receive the news: "*You have cancer*", it's truly a life threatening event. Your whole world outlook changes. This is what happened to me and to the men and women I interviewed for this book when we first heard, "You have cancer."

This book was written at the behest of my oncologist with the purpose of not only educating cancer patients and their families, but providers as well. Thus, Dr. Amy Law has contributed helpful comments and suggestions for this book to assist cancer patients, oncologists, nurses and other hospital personnel provide patients with sensitive, caring support.

As with *Changing Lanes,* my goal in writing the book is to educate, inform and assist readers to deal with a life changing event. In this case, to assist men and women, plus their families, go through the cancer experience and recovery. Profits from the sale of this book will be donated to the Cancer Society for research.

INTRODUCTIION

So you have cancer or perhaps someone you care about has contracted this insidious disease. This book tells about a personal journey of thoughts, emotions, experiences and learning's, from the initial phases of being diagnosed with cancer, through the maze of treatment options, dealing with side effects and attaining recovery. Through its pages you will get "the lowdown of what it's like" and what you can do and when to do it.

When dealing with cancer, some patients might feel they are climbing Mount Everest. Others might feel like they are climbing out from the emotional depths of personal anguish and dejection. Recovering from cancer requires you to search for your inner, unique way of maintaining a positive state of mind. By doing so, you fortify yourself to labor through the invasive procedures of testing, a physical operation, chemotherapy treatments and/or radiation. In this book, I've shared information from my personal experience, as well as including input from other cancer patients and research. There were times I desperately needed to know and understand more about my situation, but didn't quite know what questions to ask. That's why it's important to learn from others experiences, educate yourself by reading articles, books, and going on-line for information. In my search, I often stumbled on relevant information, after the time it could have eased my experience. I won't kid you and say this is easy, as there will be times you may feel "like hell". But, don't give up. If you are told you have cancer, you begin a mortal battle for your life, and you need to steel your inner self to survive it.

Whether you are the cancer victim, care giver, or medical provider, Dr. Law and I desire to share knowledge and information for a successful patient recovery experience. Let's embark on this journey of personal discovery, growth in knowledge of cancer, survival techniques and living life to the fullest in order to be the best you can be.

CHAPTER ONE

PRECANCER

Life was good in the early summer of 2012. I walked away from my doctor's office feeling pretty good about myself. After all, I had one of the best yearly physical check-ups I'd had in recent years. My husband and I retired early so we could lead active retirement lives. Over my retirement years, I exercised daily participating in activities such as: Yoga, Qi Gong, Tai Chi, land and water aerobics, walking, golf, and kayaking. My husband and I traveled on physically active vacation trips, kept busy every day involved in activities and responsibilities. We were leading the kind of life we'd hoped and planned for in our retirement years. Although, we've each had a few serious health setbacks here and there, we've been able to overcome them and carry on with our productive retirement lives.

That spring we were looking forward to a busy summer and fall. We planned to take our two grandsons on a cruise to Alaska at the end of July. In September we scheduled an active twenty-four-day trip to Greece and Turkey.

Life would have been perfect if I could just get rid of the stomach flu I was occasionally experiencing. It all started in mid-May, when I began with what might be considered a very normal health issue – an upset stomach. At first I just dismissed it as eating something that didn't agree with me. However, these symptoms continued for several weeks. This didn't seem normal. There was also a gnawing feeling in my stomach, abdominal cramps, bloating and spasms of pain in my intestines. The pain woke me up at night, and I found it difficult to get a good night's sleep. In addition, I vacillated between diarrhea and constipation for periods of time. I still thought it was some kind of flu bug or stress. At the time I had been experiencing some undue stress and considered the stress could possibly be influencing my condition. I decided to once and for all find out what was wrong. That was when I made an early yearly checkup appointment with my primary care physician. I, also, began keeping a journal of my daily food diet for about three weeks prior to the meeting. I wanted to find out what was causing my problems and perhaps eliminate those foods that may be the culprits.

The yearly checkup and tests resulted in positive numbers - blood pressure, electrolytes, kidney, blood sugar, liver function, blood count thyroid, LDL and HDL were all very good. The only issues were my Vitamin D was a little low. Thus, it seemed that all health signs were a confirmation that I was okay and doing the right things. I felt positive and safe. I assured myself that nothing could be wrong, but vowed not to eat spicy foods or difficult foods to digest for a while.

That summer we did travel with grandchildren to Alaska, seeing the sights, going on small hikes, walking on glaciers, exercising every day on the ship.

In September we actively toured Greece doing short hikes and climbing up multiple stairs to Greek monasteries. We continued our trip on a cruise of the Greek Isles and a tour of Turkey and Cappadocia climbing around ancient ruins and trekking through cave dwellings. All through the trip, I was careful not to eat very spicy foods or foods that may be difficult to digest. I, also, limited drinking wine or alcoholic beverages. I watched my diet and appeared to have no problems. Upon returning home, I continued to eat light meals, cereal or eggs for breakfast, soups for lunch and fish of chicken for dinner. I switched to Lactaid milk, and cut down drinking decaf coffee and tea. Everything seemed to be okay.

Then in November, we visited our son and daughter-in-law's home for Thanksgiving. We celebrated by partaking of a traditional, turkey dinner. Still being leery of upsetting my stomach, I ate very small portions, of turkey, dressing, cranberry sauce, vegetable and a sliver of pumpkin pie. However, my cautious eating didn't do me any good. I spent a restless, sleepless, agonizing night of what I assumed were stomach ache pains. Taking antacids or stomach settlers in the morning helped me a little and I appeared to recover. However, when I returned home, I again made an appointment with my primary care doctor. Due to a busy schedule, she could not see me until the following week. However, I felt so sick and miserable during the weekend before my appointment, my husband insisted I go to Urgent Care. Since it was a weekend, they could not do CT Scans, but did take a blood sample and took an X-ray. I received an antibiotic shot and was encouraged to obtain more tests when I saw my doctor.

My primary care doctor was able to access the X-ray results, gave me a physical checkup, and was concerned about a thickening of an area in my stomach. She referred me for a blood test and further assessments from my gastroenterologist. I thought I would have some procedure the next week. However, I was told I had to first have an office appointment. A week and one-half later I met him in his office. He wanted me to have a colonoscopy and endoscopy. I asked, "Is the colonoscopy really necessary? I had a clean colonoscopy just three years ago." He responded, "Yes" and set up the procedures for eight days later. It was getting close to Christmas, and I was getting nervous, as we were due to fly up to Portland, Oregon to visit our other son and family. The day after the tests, the gastroenterologist telephoned me to share his suppositions with me. He said, "You have cancer. We believe the cancer may have begun in your stomach and spread to your colon." As I listened to his voice over the phone, I was physically shaking, and I literally felt like I was dropping down, down, down through a sinkhole in the floor. Oh my God, how could this happen? Cancer doesn't run in my family. They die from strokes. Needless to say his news was shocking and completely overwhelmed me. As his words sunk in, I had the sense the grim reaper was calling me. Thoughts raced through my mind. If the cancer had metastasized from my stomach to my colon, it must be far advanced. How could this be? I eat well, exercise, never smoked, have had clean on-going colonoscopy assessments. After what seemed like an eternity, I was finally able to utter a question, "Can I still fly to Portland for Christmas?" He said, "Yes, as nothing could be done over the holiday."

So, my husband and I flew to Portland for the Christmas holiday. However, it didn't feel anything like our usual joyous family holidays. I shared my diagnosis with our sons and families. Both families were surprised and expressed concern and support. It was difficult for me not to let my diagnosis affect how I felt, although I tried not to show how scared and broken hearted I felt at the time. I attempted to keep these feelings to myself, and I put on a brave face for my family. I didn't want to totally spoil Christmas for them. In addition to these personal feelings, and not knowing what was to come, I realized I had to cancel part-time professional teaching commitments I had made for the winter semester at our local college.

While deep inside I felt the impinging threat of death hanging over me, I somehow pulled myself together. I said to myself, "Okay, you have now been diagnosed – now what?"

Learning's:

- The majority of cancer cases are a result of environment, aging, diet and exercise. But, family history and lifestyle do affect cancer risk.
- To be aware of your body and any changes in health that last more than a few weeks. Don't put off getting noted changes medically checked.
- Not to assume I was safe just because I got all the basic cancer screenings, never smoked, protected myself from sun exposure,

limited alcohol consumption, exercised regularly, controlled my weight and ate healthy. I perhaps lulled myself into thinking I wasn't a candidate for cancer.

- Five-to-ten percent of cancer cases relate to family genetic changes. However, behaviors and other risk factors are still being studied. Initially, when I received my cancer diagnosis, I was surprised. I didn't think cancer ran in my family. During the months after my original diagnosis, I researched and acquired further information which showed my father's side of the family did have cancer issues going back two generations.

- You need to take steps to educate yourself about your type of cancer and what can be done about it. This will be a step-by-step process based on your personal need to know. Seeking information from the American Cancer Society, on-line, in books, AARP articles, Cancer sites and Cancer magazines provided me with a perspective on addressing some of the common concerns, managing information, and finding out what I needed to know so I could make knowledgeable decisions in my cancer journey.

Surviving: A Colon Cancer Diary

CHAPTER TW0

NEXT STEP - AFTER DIAGNOSIS

Upon returning home from the family Christmas holiday, my brain was wrapped around the threat cancer posed for me. I felt death was staring me in the face. My life could shortly be over. It was too soon! All kinds of thoughts rushed through my head. I wasn't ready for this. I may likely have just a small amount of time left on this earth. When Erma Bombeck, the noted author and humorist, was told she would die from cancer, she wrote a piece entitled, "If I Had My Life to Live Over". It listed many personal experiences she remembered, and wished she had paid more attention to at the time. I, too, experienced a similar feeling of possible loss. I asked myself: Why didn't I finish those memoirs for family? Why haven't we spent more time together? Why have I wasted time on other inconsequential activities? How much time will I have with my loved ones? All kinds of thoughts raced through my brain. What would I want to be said in an obituary? Believe it or not, I did draft an obit on my computer. I read somewhere that a cancer diagnosis brings uncertainty and questions into one's life. It's not unusual to feel a little out of control initially. It's hard to remember this, when you are the one getting the cancer diagnosis and sensing a loss of control.

The first week in January, 2013 things began to move quickly. A battery of tests began. First, I went through a gastrointestinal endoscopy procedure. The report suggested I had a non-bleeding gastric ulcer, which appeared noncancerous. Wow! A sense of relief rushed through me! One issue may be resolved. It's probably only a gastric ulcer. But, then I received the news my right colon, as initially forecast, actually did have an adenocarcinoma tumor.

I next went through what one could call a "limbo" time of unknowing. I felt as if I was functioning in the dark. I kept saying to myself that if only I could emotionally back away from my situation and educate myself; I'd be able to make better, clearer, logical decisions. But, when you have life threatening cancer hanging over you, your sense of trying anything to get rid of it kicks into high gear. As a patient, you wade through the mountains of information, tests, test results, medical lingo about antibodies, curative therapy, palliative therapy, and tumor marker tests. You can feel lost and just struggle to understand. That is why I've included educational learning information at the end of each chapter in this book. To help others learn early on what I learned along the way.

Early on in my process a combination PET/CT* scan was conducted. Of course, I received copies of the reports. But, reading medical reports is like reading Latin or Greek. It's a new lexicon or language, in an unfamiliar field. *"There is intense activity demonstrated within the distal ascending colon involving the proximal hepatic flexure area......"* You need a medical dictionary to help you understand your own medical condition, unless you are medically trained or oriented. However, I was able to discern from the radiologist's impression that the cancer may not have spread from the colon. His assessment read: "*High-grade activity within biopsy-proven distal ascending colon carcinoma. No abnormal uptake in the stomach to correspond with known gastric ulcer. It is noted that the colon carcinoma and area of interest in the distal gastric body are remote from each other and believed unrelated.*"

When experiencing cancer and the threat of dying, you are thankful for every bit of positive news that comes your way. I focused on stepping back, however slightly, from my emotional fear, to view the medical process as my route to overcoming cancer and the procedures became somewhat more acceptable to me.

After all, my main goal was to find a way to get rid of the cancer. I wanted to locate an antidote or try anything to get rid of it and needed to find out if the colon cancer was operable. I found I had to back away mentally from my emotional involvement in the process to look at my situation more clearly. I needed to view the information logically. Many of us, diagnosed with cancer, may find it difficult to go through extensive testing or having to plough through mountains of information, tests and results. If you are afraid of going through medical tests, you can take comfort that you are not alone. There are many people that feel the same way. I think what we have to keep in the front of our minds is that the diagnostic procedures and tests are designed to help the professionals locate our problem and determine the best treatment plan. It was reassuring to me when a health care professional explained what would be happening in the procedure and why it was necessary. I even felt reassured when I was updated during a long procedure. There are patients who may not want to know what is going on, and they should make their preference known. However, I found by educating myself about the testing and monitoring process, I felt I could somewhat control the emotional aspect of my situation and make clear and logical decisions. I won't kid you it was very difficult as I was living this process emotionally and physically.

Learning's:

- The most effective tool to guide you through cancer recovery is KNOWLEDGE.
- Search for information on-line by accessing GOOGLE or YAHOO, The

Beverly A. Battaglia, Ph.D

American Cancer Society, Mayo Clinic. Just put in the topic you are researching.
- Check AMAZON, book stores, libraries for recent books on your type of cancer.
- On-line check other sites such as: guide2Chemo.com or
- www.Caring4Cancer.com.
- Check out books and/or magazines which focus on Cancer – such as Caring4Cancer, or Guide to Chemotherapy.

CHAPTER THREE

SURGERY

Needless to say, I felt a sense of immediacy and set up several appointments: first with my primary care physician, to discuss the possibility of surgery and obtain a referral to a recommended surgeon. My husband and I met with a surgeon a few days later. Walking into his office, I experienced some trepidation about what he would say. After reviewing my up-to-date information forwarded to him, he said "Your colon cancer is operable." I was immensely relieved to hear him utter those words. They were a lifeline when I felt I was in peril of drowning. In order to make a wise decision and learn more about the kind of cancer I had, I compiled a list of questions to ask at this meeting such as: the doctor's experience with this type of operation, level of tumor penetration, surgery and recovery time, etc. His approach would be to do a full cut surgery where I would be in the hospital for 7-10 days and have 3-4 weeks of convalescence. But, now I knew I had a chance to live! My second appointment that day was with his recommended cardiologist who ran tests to see if I was physically up to such a surgery. He gave me his okay for the operation. I left the healthcare facilities feeling more relieved than I had in weeks. My colon cancer was operable.

At this point, I was getting a better handle on the situation and said "not so fast". Let me take time to research colon cancer operations and get other recommendations. In addition to obtaining a second opinion, I found there was a possibility the operation could be done laparoscopically. Immediately I went to work checking on-line for laparoscopic surgeons in our area, who specialized in colon surgery. I also obtained referrals from friends and neighbors. Two and one-half years before I had my hip replaced laparoscopically and it went extremely well. So, I was comfortable with this type of procedure. I made an appointment with a highly recommended laparoscopic surgeon in my area.

Surviving: A Colon Cancer Diary

As if I didn't have enough to worry about at this time, my sinuses decided to act up and I got an infection. Thanks to my ENT (ear nose and throat) physician, who fit me into his schedule and prescribed antibiotics, I recovered pretty quickly.

For meetings with each doctor – my primary care physician, surgeons, and those involved in my after care, I always prepared an agenda of what I had to know and questions I needed answered. This does take time and thought, but I felt it was worth it. I would highly recommend this to other patients for any of their physician appointments. Your time with your doctor is limited, you want to make the most of it and get the information you need to get and stay well.

In order to ask questions, remember you need to do some research on your condition - type of cancer, possible surgeries or treatments. Then you can ask appropriate questions to obtain the information you want. Don't be afraid to ask about how long a surgeon has been practicing or how many surgeries he/she has done. When the surgeon shares information, don't be afraid to ask follow-up questions if you aren't clear or don't understand. In my case, I asked about what is involved in laparoscopic colon surgery, tests in preparation for surgery, type of anesthetic, length of time in the hospital, home recuperation issues and what might come after surgery. In my discussion with the surgeon more questions evolved during the conversation. Here again, it helps to have someone with you to help you ask questions, or write down information. You then must rely on that person to corroborate or remember what transpired in the meeting. What I relied on most in meetings is my small portable tape recorder. I had used it for interviewing participants when writing my book, *Changing Lanes: Couples Redefining Retirement*. I would first obtain permission to tape our conversation, tape it and transcribe it that day or the next day, so I would have clear information as to what was said and prescribed. It was not only a God send because it helped me verify important directions and information, but it was a useful in later doctor appointments. Thus, I would recommend it highly, to keep information, directions, medications, and health status straight. It's amazing how your ears can deceive you or your attention span lag for a second or two when you can miss important information.

By electing laparoscopic surgery, I would only be in the hospital three days, with few weeks of convalescence at home. My only lingering concern was: could the entire cancer tumor be taken out with this operating method? However, I elected this approach and the operation date was set for two weeks later. After the surgeon's physical exam, came more tests - blood tests, another electrocardiogram EKG, urine test, chest X-rays. At this time, I was diagnosed with Stage Two cancer because the tumor appeared to be within the colon. I was given to expect I'd be in the hospital three-four days. I'd have intravenous infusions of fluids to prevent dehydration and fluid loss. No food by mouth because the intestines would be inactive. Recovery time would be one to two months where I had to follow a high fiber diet and not lift heavy objects. The surgeon said that since my tumor was in an early stage, I may not need chemotherapy. However, if the lymph nodes were infected or other cancer cells discovered, I may need chemotherapy with or without radiation per his recommendation.

After my meeting with the laparoscopic surgeon, I prepared a list of pluses and minuses for a decision meeting with my primary care physician two days later. As you can see, things were moving pretty fast. She'd been my doctor for about ten years and I felt comfortable discussing my concerns and misgivings with her. After obtaining her input, I made my decision to go ahead with the laparoscopic surgery. I then broached the subject of how to treat my stomach ulcer. What medications, vitamins, should I be taking? Also, I requested a food guide and the name of a good nutritionist to aid me. We, thus, formulated a plan to heal the stomach ulcer. At this time, I felt under enormous stress to make the right decisions, as I felt my life did depend on it. I felt reasonably comfortable as I had gotten input from my husband and my primary care physician and thus, made my decision. I was fortunate to have my husband's full support, as well as my family's support as I stepped into the "unknown".

I was operated on January 22, 2013, approximately seven weeks after first being diagnosed with cancer. I don't remember much about the operation, but still remember being surprised to get a single patient room. I also remember walking around and around the hospital hallways during the few days after the operation. The laparoscopic surgeon stopped to see me in my hospital room later on the day of my surgery. He had successfully excised the cancerous section of my colon. However, he shared that the cancerous tumor had poked through the colon wall infecting one lymph node out of the forty-three the pathologist examined. This changed my diagnosis to Stage III because lymph nodes can travel throughout the body and spread the cancer to various other organs such as the liver. This was not the news I hoped to hear, as it meant further tests and extensive treatment would be necessary. I felt somewhat downhearted when I shared this news with my husband and family later in the day.

We all have a fear of the unknown. Even the word CANCER frightens people because it can mean suffering and death. For me, as I lived through this process, pursuing information on tests for cancer, treatments and survival stories helped me to be less fearful than I felt initially. I tried to psychologically understand the medical process and lingo thrown at me such as tumor marker tests, blood counts, kinds of imaging tests, etc. As patients, we are told to ask questions about our illness or treatment, but sometimes we don't know enough about what to ask.

But, even with education, in the back of my mind was the gnawing thought of having this frightening disease called cancer. I forced myself to realize all the doctor meetings, assessments, treatments, prodding, poking, and tests are being done to help me. The question was how to steel myself to go through them and not lose faith with the process or with myself?

One and one-half weeks after my surgery some of the questions, which began to run through my head, were answered at my follow-up appointment with the surgeon. After removing my staples, he took the time to consult with my husband and me. He had collected forty-three lymph nodes and found one cancerous. I asked why he had collected so many, as the standard was generally twelve or sixteen. He explained the process was to clean out my lymph node basin and it was clear. However, chemotherapy was necessary, because there could be one or two rogue cells that may have gone to the liver or to the lung tissue. It was an unknown at the time. So, I guess I was lucky he had collected so many, for who knew if the seventeenth, or thirtieth or fortieth was the infected node? He felt that my risk was pretty small that forty-two out of forty-three lymph nodes were negative and he had done a clean resection. I was reassured to hear my surgeon say he believed I had a standard case of cancer and most likely would not need radiation. However, I would still need months of chemotherapy. So, I had a long journey ahead of me, but felt somewhat better moving out of what I call "the neutral zone" when I was unsure of where to go or what step to take next.

Learning's:

- It's important to have a good primary care physician to be your quarterback through the cancer process.
- Although I have heard others discuss the Stages of Cancer and have read a few articles in AARP or doctor's offices, I never fully understood the details dictating cancer stages, or many of the other terms related to

cancer. As a patient, I felt it imperative to take the time to research this more fully.

- In relation to cancer staging (in my case colon cancer) medical personnel refer to the amount of penetration of a specific cancer. The common staging system is the TNM or tumors/nodes/metastases system. My cancer was labeled T3.

"T" represents the degree of invasion of an intestinal wall

"N" represents the degree of lymphatic node involvement

"M" represents the degree of metastasis or spread to other organs

Stage 0   Tumor is confined to mucosa or mucous membrane

Stage 1   A small cancer is found only in the organ where it began (T1 or T2)

Stage 2   A larger cancer which may or may not spread to the lymph nodes (T3 or T4)

Stage 3   A larger cancer that has spread to the lymph nodes (T1-2 or T3-4)

Surviving: A Colon Cancer Diary

Stage 4   A cancer found in a different organ from where it began (any T)

**(Further references on Wikipedia – Colon Cancer Staging)*

Beverly A. Battaglia, Ph.D

CHAPTER FOUR

TREATMENT OPTIONS

At this point in recovery, I was one-month post-surgery and was ready for what they call Adjuvant Therapy*. I felt good and everything was healing well. I had started taking long walks and was up to about one mile a day. My appetite was okay, considering I was on medications and a bland diet because of the stomach ulcer. I had no abominable pain, no diarrhea nor constipation. I went right back to normal bowel movements once a day in the morning. Although I dropped nine pounds during the last two months, I had begun to put back on three-four pounds.

In the weeks of recuperation after my operation, I began research of treatment options and oncologists. My research consisted of talking with my primary care physician, asking friends familiar with cancer care, for oncologist references, as well as checking on my computer. By researching on the computer you cannot only assess care providers, but also see information on various doctors, their backgrounds and experience. I was determined to locate the "right" oncologist for me. I discussed the various experiences people had, as well as the doctor's professional reputation, personality and bedside manner. I foresaw the months ahead of me would most likely to be difficult, and I wanted the best care I could get. I also spent time assessing the reputations of hospitals and oncology medical groups.

I might mention here, that over the years I had prepared a number of documents. One was an end-of-life treatment document on file with my primary care physician and local hospital. The other two documents are information lists that I share with new physicians. One is a list of all my past surgeries, doctors with addresses and phone numbers. The second list is of all the medications and vitamin supplements I take. Each list has to be updated yearly if changes occur. Sharing these lists can speed things up when checking in with a new physician or surgeon.

My first meeting was with a local recommended oncologist. The agenda was to discuss my condition, what recovery approach the oncologist would take and what that process would be like. She agreed I had a fairly straight forward type of Stage III cancer and took time to explain her chemotherapy approach. Her protocol would include a regimen of two chamoes together. One is 5-FU, an oral chemotherapy drug called Xeloda and an intravenous 5-FU called Oxaliplatin. The intravenous drug could be provided in one of two ways. First, it could be delivered through a personally operated chemo pump requiring infusion over 44 hours through an injection. The second was through a mediport catheter. The mediport catheter would need to be surgically inserted into my upper chest. With the mediport method I would spend 3 – 3 ½ hours every three weeks to have the chemo drug drip into my vein through the catheter.

The oncologist took time to explain the pathology report. She suggested standardized treatment and answered many of my questions. Because I had read somewhere that it is important to be aware of the latest treatments, I asked about possible clinical studies on Stage

III cancer patients. I was told that of the studies she was aware of, focused on stage IV patients and clinical studies hadn't shown new drugs helping Stage III patients.

The definition of cure is that I would be cancer free for five consecutive years from the day I had surgery. If I am cancer free in January 2018, I'll be told I am cured. When I began chemo, if I had surgery alone, knowing it involved one cancerous lymph node, my chance of being cured was roughly 50%. What oncologists know for a fact after two decades of practice is that the addition of chemotherapy treatment following surgery improves a patient's cure rate by an additional 10% or a cure percentage of 60%. In other words, chemotherapy treatment will reduce my chance of cancer coming back about from 50% to 40%. That may not sound highly optimistic, as it didn't to me when I first heard it, but the only time a doctor can say cancer is 100% gone is when the patient never contracted cancer in the first place. The oncologist was very open and shared detailed information on medications, side effects, and chemo's effect on my stomach ulcer condition.

Beverly A. Battaglia, Ph.D

Although I received a lot of helpful information and was satisfied with the meeting, I still felt I needed to learn more and check other recommended oncologists to see if they might have a different approach for my recovery. Since a patient has the right to a second opinion, I obtained an okay from Medicare for another opinion from an oncologist at the third highest rated cancer care provider in the United States.

The doctor's location was some 150 miles from my home, which could make it difficult to travel every few weeks for treatment. This meeting, with the university oncologist, continued to enlighten both my husband and me about my cancer treatment options. With each oncologist meeting, we became more aware and educated, so we were able to ask more in depth questions. Initially, we were told about 150,000 people a year get colon cancer in this country. So, fairly basic protocols have been established and accepted as being standard. He said that they would no longer be treating my active cancer, but would be focusing on the possibility that there might be some microscopic cells, not visible on a CAT scan and not visible in pathology, that might have squeezed their way out and are circulating in my body. They could be the source of a problem two to three years out. This doctor thought the pathologist did a good job checking 43 lymph nodes, as his university center generally checks a lower number. This doctor verified the standard of care at stage III rectal colon cancer is the use of the two chemo drugs (5-FU Oxaliplatin and oral version of 5-FU Xeloda) together. However, he shared a recent study that questioned the benefit of Oxaliplatin infusions for patients my age (70's). There were pros and cons as to the added benefit of both to me. My option could be to have an IV shot once and see how I react, but he thought it much more important that I go with the 5-FU pill. Usually this oncologist treats a patient for six months and then reassesses at that time. After that, assessments are done every three to six months going forward for the next few years. I was reassured that the chemotherapy most likely won't make my stomach ulcer dramatically worse. So, I came away from this meeting with greater understanding of the recovery process, but with questions about the varied approach to treatment.

In order to determine a specific treatment plan from the two slightly diverse opinions, I was allowed to get a third opinion. So, I made an appointment at another well-known cancer care center about two hours from where we live.

At this meeting, the oncologist said a good surgery is anything above twelve lymph nodes collected and he thought forty-three was very good. The treatment plan at this facility slightly differed from the first and second oncologists' treatment plans. They would provide an infusion method called Folfox, or Capox infusion of Oxaliplatin plus pill every two weeks for twelve times. Either way I would need to have a port inserted in my chest. This oncologist felt that his way or the first oncologist's method was good.

One differing point he made was he doesn't use a PET scan for surveillance of a patient because his hospital doesn't want to expose the patient to too much radiation with a lot of scans. The concern was a higher chance of secondary cancer due to too much radiation. They usually do a CAT scan after surgery to use as a baseline. I asked if treatment is usually begun within six weeks of surgery, and was told it's begun as close to surgery as possible, once the patient recovers. The rational is that if a small cell was left behind in the body, which can't be seen, it can divide one to two to four, four to eight, so the longer a patient has to wait; it defeats the purpose of obtaining preventative medications. This information instilled in me a sense of urgency to make a decision and proceed with the chemotherapy as soon as possible.

I, also, found out that his facility did have clinical trials going on at the time, but only on patients who did not have their tumor break through the colon wall. So, I would not be a candidate for trials. I thanked the oncologist for his information and we left. I now had sufficient information to base a knowledgeable decision on. I realized I'd better make my decision promptly.

Having learned so much more about chemotherapy from the interview meetings with the oncologists, I could ask more clear and specific questions about the process and its affects. I still had questions about the Mediport insertion and the two-fold process of fighting any rogue cancer cells.

I utilized my follow-up appointment with the laparoscopic surgeon to ask a few more questions and obtain his views, based on his experience. I taped our conversation and ended up with six double-spaced pages of detailed answers to my questions.

Here are the relevant, informational points I learned from the taped conversations I had with the three oncologists and the laparoscopic surgeon.

- I received assurance that my lymph node base was clear and I had a clean colon resection – thus making my risk pretty small.
- Chemotherapy was necessary as an attempt to kill the one or two rogue cells which may have spread somewhere else in my body.
- The chance of recurrence would be smaller if I went ahead with chemotherapy as soon as possible.
- There are several levels of chemotherapy I could have:

A. Take only the 5-FU Xeloda pills – because of my low risk factor one lymph node infected out of forty-three.

B. The multiagent therapy of infusion chemotherapy – Folfox type (Oxaliplatin and 5-FU Xeloda) multiagent treatment is more aggressive with more side effects and possibly more complications. It is likely to be more effective for long term cancer cure.

It was up to me to weigh the high amount of toxicity I was willing to accept getting the infusion chemotherapy plus Xeloda pills or go with the lower toxicity 5-FU Xeloda pills, with fewer side effects and was tolerated by most patients. The question was: would this approach be effective for me? Did I want to take that chance? There may be a study out that states the two-prong approach wasn't necessary for patients my age, but, as a non-medical professional, did I want to take this critical time to delve into what the studies showed to determine what specific study results showed for people my age? I opted not to do further research and decided to go with the two-prong, Folfox Type of chemotherapy.

Although I discussed the treatment pluses and minuses with my husband, I was the one who had to decide on treatment. It was my health and my life. I had to make a decision and live with the consequences. If I went through the treatment and got a massive bleeding ulcer because of it, I'd most likely kick myself and say "I should have taken the milder approach." But, if I'd taken the milder approach and had a recurrence of my cancer three years down the road, I'd say, "I should have taken the more stringent approach."

At home, after transcribing all my notes from each of the meetings, and assessing the approaches to treatment, I decided that the best approach for me would be to go with an oncologist who would use both methods of chemotherapy. I'd been a little skeptical about utilizing only chemo pills, and felt we needed to do everything possible, to figuratively "throw the book at it" type of approach in my cancer battle. However, I was glad I had taken the time and effort to collect detailed information on the process. It was reassuring to me to hear my surgeon believe I could physically withstand the two-pronged approach if need be. Given my own personal needs and temperament, I felt most comfortable in going to the local oncologist, who was recommended to me. She was not only knowledgeable but seemed to bring a connective, caring, approach to her work with patients. I went with Dr. Amy Law.

Learning's:

- In order to make an informed decision as to treatment of cancer, the patient and/or advocate needs to research and read up on the various options. Unfortunately, there is little time available as a decision needs to be made in a short time.
- Don't be afraid to obtain second opinions and other medical approaches.
- Select an oncologist you feel comfortable with as he or she will be your support and guide in your cancer battle.

Beverly A. Battaglia, Ph.D

CHAPTER FIVE

TREATMENT BEGINS

The first step in beginning the treatment phase of cancer recovery was to have a PET scan. It was done after my operation to provide a pictorial basis for further initial treatment. The second step in beginning my two-pronged treatment plan was to have a mediport inserted. So, five weeks after my colon surgery, I met with the surgeon to find out what was involved in inserting the mediport and educate myself as to any issues or possible repercussions.

I was told the mediport catheter would be the chemotherapy access that is inserted under the skin beneath the clavicle bones. You can see it through the skin, but it is underneath. It sticks out enough so that chemotherapy nurses can find it and poke a needle into it. The chemo medication is not inserted directly into a patient's veins, because over time, the process can trash the veins. The mediport allows medical professionals to draw blood easily and allows for the infusion of the chemotherapy toxic chemicals into the patient's vascular system through the mechanical device which is connected to the patient's subclaving vein (one that goes out to the arm). I asked, "Just what is it?" The surgeon said it is a piece of plastic in a vein. There sometimes are potential problems in getting it inserted, and he has to be careful not to pop a lung as the site is near a patient's lung. He mentioned that mediports can get infected, and I'd need to be careful who accesses the port. The oncologist nurses take care of the ports as they need to be cleaned properly and kept very sterile. Apparently mediports could experience several complications, but I was assured that these could be dealt with during treatment. A mechanical malfunction could occur such as the catheter twisting around, or breaking. But I was told most of the time this doesn't happen and most patients are fine. Perhaps 2 – 3 percent of people have a problem with their mediport and the surgeon said it could be dealt with. I asked, "How long does a port stay in when treatment is completed?" I was told that it is left in as long as treatment is going on and for a reasonable time afterwards. Typically, if the patient is cured, the port can be taken out.

The mediport will be inserted on the left side of my chest in a one-half hour surgery at a day surgery center. I will have a dressing over the surgery and will have to follow-up with oncology nurses within one week after surgery. My first chemotherapy appointment was to be within a week of the insertion, so I was told they would teach me more about port operation. The nurses apparently take ownership of the port, even though it is in my body. At the time it sounded like a relief to me.

I asked the surgeon if there was a way to determine risk of recurrence of cancer since it's probably different with each patient treated. I was told that all doctors have is the pathology and that the biology of a tumor isn't well understood and somewhat unknown. I guess the pathology will dictate what happens to me in the next five years. What I know is that chemotherapy improves your survival grossly by ten percent for stage IIIB. So I get a gross 30% improvement in five-year survival rate.

Although I had hoped for a greater percentage, I had to accept the facts.

Chemotherapy #1 - March 7, 2013

My next step was the first meeting with my oncologist prior to my chemotherapy. A nurse weighed me and took a blood sample to determine if I met the criteria to go ahead with chemotherapy. The doctor reviewed my recent PET scan which showed two small metabolic foci (lesions) in the right lobe of my liver, which was a little disconcerting so soon in my therapy, because it could mean early metastases (the cancer had spread). I wrote down SCARY in my meeting notes. But, I'd have to wait to find out. My doctor was going to obtain another radiologist's opinion. Otherwise everything else appeared within reason, given my recent surgery.

I was told I had a favorable type of colon cancer, which allows for more treatment options. I thought at the time what a strange combination of words, "favorable cancer". Apparently this "favorable cancer" opened up a lot treatment options for me. My doctor recommended Capox infusion every three weeks and chemotherapy pills two weeks on and one week off. She felt Capox was more convenient for her patients. She also suggested taking Nexium and Calcium carbonate 2-3 times a day...to address my ulcer and raise my calcium level as well. She arranged for me to meet with a nutritionist at our local hospital. This was important because the chemo could irritate my gastric ulcer. We went over various medications to help me once I begin the chemo pills.

In addition, we discussed expected infusion reactions I might experience. One is the extreme sensitivity to cold especially the first two days after treatment – avoid cold drinks or drinks with ice, no ice packs, no deep breathing in cold air or air conditioning, and no going into the refrigerator. There were thirteen possible side effects from the chemotherapy infusion and pills. I thought it important to list some those that affected me.

- Fatigue – which builds with each additional chemotherapy treatment
- Neuropathy – numbness, tingling, prickling, dulled sensation, loss of balance, walking problems, clumsiness,

difficulty picking up small objects or buttoning clothing
- Diarrhea and nausea
- Constipation
- Loss or change of appetite
- Aversion to cold temperatures, cold drinks, ice, cold objects

My oncologist assured me that I would get through the treatment and be able to deal with the side effects. She suggested that once I got control of the side effects, my experience would actually be easier than raising my children.

I went in for my first chemotherapy infusion after this meeting. At 10:30 a.m. I entered a long, bright, sunny room with lounge chairs along each side. Light streamed through the windows along one side. The windows faced out on to Mount San Jacinto. As I walked in, I made a mental note to select a vacant lounge chair which faced the mountains. I noted number of patients of various ages being given their chemotherapy through bags hanging from steel stilts. There were approximately five or six nurses working with the different patients. I was asked to select a lounge chair and selected one facing the mountains. After I made myself comfortable and sat in the chair for about twenty minutes, the nurse had received my chemo bags and was ready to connect me through my mediport to the hanging bags of chemicals. I had come prepared with a lap robe to keep me warm, plus my iPod, reading material, some juice and snacks, as I'd be here for three plus hours over lunch time. My husband came to pick me up around 2:00, as I could not drive to or from the chemo treatments. I left chemotherapy armed with instructions and a list of pills to deal with the chemo side effects: anti-nausea, vomiting, constipation, mouth sores, fatigue and instructions for medicinal helps. However, I didn't feel too limited, as I understood I could have a pedicure, massage and hair coloring during the months ahead. I decided against having a massage or a body scrub, with a port located in my upper chest, so I nixed that off my list. Given this was my first treatment; I had a follow-up two weeks later to be sure everything was going as planned.

Learning's:

- What I learned is that even though there are studies going on, the standard cancer care is driven by protocol, because doctors decided that it works and it's become the standard of care. Study groups are for trying to figure out if using new approaches is of benefit; that's the whole idea of trials.
- Prior to beginning chemo, a patient needs to take care of any dental work and get any specific exams that are due.
- Prior to beginning chemo, it helps a patient to fill all necessary prescriptions and obtain specific vitamins that are prescribed by their oncologist.
- It's easier for a woman to wear a camisole for therapy, as it provides easier access to the port opening. I wore an open button-down shirt over the camisole.
- I learned through reading and talking with other cancer survivors what paraphernalia to bring for the chemotherapy sessions: a lap warmer, a cool pack with juice, fruit, energy bar or peanut butter and crackers, sandwich and something to occupy your mind. Experienced chemotherapy patients brought magazines,

books, Kindles or Nooks, iPads, sandwiches, snacks, fruits and drinks. Some read, some conversed, some slept and others played games on their cell phones or iPads.

- To combat the sensitivity to anything cold, it helped to keep items a patient might want in the refrigerator door and to use gloves to pick it up quickly.
- I appreciated being in touch with my oncologist by email. As so often happens a patient forgets to ask a question, clarify instructions or encounters issues or problems between treatments. It's easy not to be able to think of or ask the right questions in a doctor meeting. But, once I returned home, and had researched the issue, I had more questions.
- Also, emails provided me a way to clarify something said in our meeting or follow up a commitment. My doctor usually got back to me within a day or so.

CHAPTER SIX

TREATMENT ISSUES

Chemotherapy #2 - March 28, 2013

My second chemotherapy meeting with my oncologist was two weeks after my chemo appointment. I had a CT scan done the day before, which found that my ulcer was resolved. Yea!! Something to celebrate! However, the results showed a new area of my liver affected. The radiologist found a fourth lesion, thought to be suspicious. What ran through my mind was: *Oh no, the lesions seem to have increased from the previous scan!* Apparently, when a radiologist sees increasing lesions in a cancer patient, he or she believes it to be suspicious. The easiest way to find out was to have a CT guided biopsy done in outpatient radiology. My oncologist thought it important for us to know if it was cancer or not. If it wasn't cancer, I'd remain at Stage III. If the lesions were cancerous, my condition would change to Stage IV." Dr. Law, said, "In a way I'm glad we did this PET scan, even knowing you had a PET scan before surgery. Otherwise we may not have caught the change." I then had another blood test to be sure my blood hadn't thinned with the chemo, so I wouldn't bleed during the biopsy.

The rest of the meeting focused on a discussion of side effects, vitamin supplements and exercising, and what I could do and shouldn't do. But it was difficult for me to concentrate on the meeting. I was told I had no restrictions and could do water aerobics, yoga, Qi Gong, Tai Chi, etc. However, I heard for the very first time that I should not put my left arm above my head because patients had been known to flip the catheter by raising the arm on the side where the catheter was located. I really didn't know how I was going to do water aerobics, yoga or other exercises most of which call for raising one's arms. Dr. Law said she didn't want me to be a "couch potato", but I needed to pace myself and build in time to rest. I thought at the time, that if I couldn't do most of my exercise activities, I would become a "couch potato". However, my husband expressed a concern I might overdo exercise. The doctor did caution me not to overdo. I left the office, wondering just what exercise routines were left that I could do. I was probably left with taking very long walks. I actually enjoyed walking around our community. Sometimes I walked listening to music on my iPod or I'd call different friends and we'd do what I called a "Walk-Talk". We, not only moved our feet, but our mouths as well while we caught up on events in our lives. This was a wonderful outlet for me during recovery.

Upon leaving my doctor's office I was concerned about the "raising the arm" issue, since I had already been doing Tai Chi and Yoga for a number of weeks. I decided to email her and ask if I needed another port checkup before my next chemo. My doctor answered that no port study was necessary, and there was a protocol established which nurses will follow at my next chemo therapy. I also wanted some clarification on the radiologist's report, and what assurance did I have of no cancer, if only the most recent lesion would be biopsied. I was told the radiologist would review the PET scan and determine the sampling. My medical saga continued.

    I went to the hospital radiology and was physically prepared for the biopsy. However, after I was on the table in radiology, the procedure was aborted. The radiologist decided he could not do a good biopsy because he was not able to see the lesion clearly. He wanted another MRI, so he could find the direct path to do the biopsy. There was more verbiage about not being able to get it right, a possibility of bleeding and not mudding up the waters for an MRI. But, I was disappointed and spent all that time in the procedure to no benefit. Was I receiving a professional medical run around? I also was further concerned because another MRI meant more exposure to radiation (which has been shown to lead to cancer).

    Here was another opportunity for learning. Things don't always work out the way it was planned. Disappointments and changes would happen, and I just had to adjust to them, if I had no control. This might be one of the more difficult learning's; *you are not in control of your body's recovery process.*

Surviving: A Colon Cancer Diary

In the pre-chemo meeting with the oncologist, we not only covered the MRI/biopsy issue, but went over my stats and progress. I was to go through twelve cycles of chemotherapy scheduled to last over eight months. I found out that sitting in the sun can cause my skin to burn, and it was important to use sun screen. I reported that I was feeling somewhat tired but seemed to tolerate the first chemo reasonably well. With this chemo treatment, I would be two down and ten to go. It seemed like a long journey.

Three days later, I had the MRI and received a call from my oncologist. She reported that the MRI showed three liver lesions. Where was the fourth? The biopsy was scheduled the next week. The radiologist would attempt to get four samples and he would have a pathologist in the operating room to check immediately with a microscope.

As a patient you can feel like a Guiney pig – being poked, screened, scanned, weighed, and needled. The process becomes a jumble of white blood cells, platelets, metabolic panels, X-rays, CAT scans, and PET scans. One can feel overwhelmed, while all the time in the back of your mind is the gnawing thought – I have this frightening disease called cancer. How can I get rid of it? You mentally understand all these doctor meetings, treatments, prodding, poking, and tests are supposed to help you. The question is how to steel yourself to go through them and not lose faith in the process, in the doctors and in yourself? The next week I checked into the hospital and went down to the Special Procedures department for the liver biopsy. I met the same technical staff and greeted each by name. But, it wasn't old friend's week.

Chemotherapy #3 - April 18, 2013

At my next oncology appointment, I received excellent news that the liver biopsy showed no evidence of cancer. The lesions were just scars on my liver. Yes, I heaved a big sigh of relief. The cancer hadn't metastasized. Another issue circumvented.

After noting my puffy, itchy eyes, Dr. Law prescribed a new eye drop medicine, which might help me. The doctor asked about my energy level. Although I was experiencing more tiredness, I was still able to present two seminars based on my retirement book at a recent conference. Apparently the third week after receiving chemo, I experienced a resurgence of energy right before my next treatment. However, after a number of treatments, my energy level continued to go down, but the fatigue was manageable. I allowed myself some time to rest during the day. Sometimes I would sit and read, or watch TV. I read that walking helps renew energy when feeling fatigued. When I did walk, I actually felt better and had a little more energy.

At this point in the conversation, my husband said, "I have to slow her down." Dr. Law suggested that life was not a marathon, and I should pace myself and not sprint through my recovery. However, I didn't feel I was sprinting or overdoing. I'm a naturally active person. At this time, Dr. Law shared what she saw as the natural psychology of a cancer patient going though treatment. The minute they begin to feel better, they believe that they have the energy to do everything. Then, they crash and burn and wonder why. Because of this, my doctor suggested taking one thing at a time and prioritizing chores. This chemo session would total three treatments down and nine to go.

I was getting used to the chemotherapy room routine and began to know all the nurses by first name. I became acquainted with several of the patients that came for treatment on my same day and time. Often, patients would bring in cookies and candy for the staff. It was a special cookie occasion when a patient had their last chemo and graduated.

Chemotherapy #4 - May 9, 2013

Dr. Law first took her assessment of my condition: tiredness - no, mouth sores-no, diarrhea - no, etc. I reported being more tired after the last round of chemo and had a numbing sensitivity in my fingers, palms and soles of my feet. However, I was able to write with a pen and could still work on the computer with no problem. The cold sensitivity continued for the first two or three days after treatment. My son recently watched me get something from the refrigerator while wearing my winter gloves and laughingly asked if I was going to put on a parka, too! Generally, I wasn't experiencing any major changes. I had a more overactive bladder for about two weeks after my infusion and wondered if it was related to chemo treatment. Doctor said most patients get neuropathy in their hands and feet. She hypothesized that perhaps the nerve ending issues to the bladder could contribute to having to pee more often. I was also experiencing an unsettled stomach, perhaps nausea. Doctor suggested Tums or Maalox might help. She said, "Most patients find that as chemo treatments go on, it's a lot less upsetting to the stomach if you eat small frequent meals rather than sitting down to traditional breakfast, lunch and dinner portions." I mentioned that I have been eating salad plate portions and tried to have snacks or an energy bar between meals. At this time, I received my mammogram checkup notice, and my doctor suggested I wait with that, given the mediport placement. She said the chemo pills would take care of things.

I mentioned that I had tried a light session of water aerobics. She stated I didn't have to feel cocooned or sheltered, when going through chemotherapy. I should feel confident to lead as normal a life as I can. "Just follow common sense." At the time I wondered if my common sense was the same as my doctor's definition of common sense. In Chemotherapy sessions, I was four down, eight to go.

My chemotherapy treatment was not going as smoothly as it had originally. My sessions were taking more time than previously. The port didn't seem to be functioning properly and needed to be flushed to open it up to take the chemo.

About this time, I checked with my doctor about driving to northern California for an aunt's 90th birthday party. She said no problem. Since we'd be in northern California, we planned a mini-vacation of two or three days in San Francisco. My husband felt I needed a break from the rounds of doctors, illness and chemo treatments. However, after attending the party, I became very ill that night with an upset stomach and diarrhea which lasted thirty-six hours. I was miserable. It was difficult being so ill in a motel room with my husband running to and from the local pharmacy. What helped were Imodium D and Gatorade. We decided to cancel the San Francisco stay and do it another time. We sadly headed back driving down the coast – home.

Chemotherapy #5 - May 30, 2013

At my next session with my oncologist, I discussed my illness on the above trip, along with my cold sensitivity lasting one and one-half weeks, rather than just three days after chemo. She verified that the Imodium worked and gave me directions about what to do if it happened again. I shared that I was using recipes from a cancer cookbook entitled, *Eating Well Through Cancer*, to help me deal with some of my physical side effects such as nausea.

Since I was experiencing further neuropathy in my hands as well as my feet, my doctor decided to lower my dose of Xelaplatin and reduce my dose of chemotherapy pills by varying the weeks I would take the pill. She explained this is why she sees me every round of treatment to evaluate the side effects and to make changes. Apparently, this is the point in chemotherapy treatment when most of her patients have cumulative neuropathy from the Xelaplatin which requires a reduction. So I was on par with her other patients. I received an okay to have needed dental filling and was told to drink more water and liquids as my sodium chloride showed low in the blood work assessment.

    My session in the chemotherapy room again took much longer than the norm. Problems arose with the slowness of the drip into my port. When I looked to the right it tended to drip. If I looked to the left, it stopped. If I looked up to see if it was dripping, it stopped, and I had to contact the nurse who would flush it out and get it to function again. Two male chemo patients in lounge chairs across from me would signal me when they saw it stop. The nurse would come over to adjust it. A few minutes later, they signaled another stoppage. It didn't matter how I moved my head or tried not to move at all, the drip stopped. It was like a comic opera. But, it wasn't funny for me or the nurse involved in constantly adjusting it. The ordeal was completed after four hours. I said we have to do something about this port problem. So, Dr. Law arranged for a port study to be done at our local hospital.

CHAPTER SEVEN

THE PORT PROBLEM

As I looked over my notes from my first meetings with my oncologist and my mediport surgeon, I did see that they mentioned treatment side effects and the surgeon defined a few of the issues a small percentage of patients could have with a mediport. But, as a patient, I was in a mindset of: "I have to do everything I can to not get cancer from those few lymph nodes." "It won't happen to me." Even reading information on-line didn't deter me, because I'd be one of the percentage of patients who didn't have a problem. Actually, I didn't see any other options available to me, other than the mediport. Unfortunately, after the first five chemotherapy treatments, I experienced what my doctor called a "non-functioning port".

Beverly A. Battaglia, Ph.D

I personally learned when a cancer patient goes through chemotherapy, he or she must call on his or her positive reserves many times because problems and issues do arise and tend to weigh you down. If you don't use the positive reserve, you can easily sink into a depressive state because you might run into what seems like one problem after another. You have to constantly reenergize yourself to think positively that you will conquer the problems that arise. Ways to help you to stay confident are practices such as meditation, positive thinking, and proactive actions.

My next mediport study showed a port blockage. So, two weeks later found me again in radiological special procedures department at the hospital. I went through a radiological procedure, which ended up lasting six hours from prep start to finish, at which time I had to lie flat on my back for a period of time after the procedure. During the procedure itself, I lay on the table, covered and blocked so I couldn't view what was happening. The radiologist gave me a shot? Then a wire was sent up through my body to the port area located above my left breast. The goal was to uncoil the tube or catheter seen on an imaging device. When he couldn't do it with one wire, a second wire riddled its way up through my body, while I listened to the professionals discuss various ways to deal with the situation. Let me say, neither wire procedure hurt in any way. It just felt strange feeling it wriggle within my body. They found the end of the catheter was jammed into the wall of the vein, like the end of a hose up against a wall. No wonder the chemotherapies were such trouble and taking so long. Back to the experience...It was actually surreal. My way of dealing with the tension of the situation was to focus my mind on something else. I imagined I was doing my tai chi exercises and that occupied my mind. At times I used positive thinking and visualization. I visualized the wire pulling the catheter away from the wall. Finally, the radiologist announced success. It was finally free. If I wasn't strapped on the table, I would have jumped with joy!

My doctor and I discussed my port experience at my next regular chemotherapy meeting. I was still concerned I may have done some exercise or movement that caused the catheter to malfunction. If so, I didn't want to do it again. We reviewed the exercises I did and could continue doing, as long as I didn't put my arm above my head. In my consulting business I spent many years solving problems for clients. My mind naturally functions in a problem solving mode. Thus, I tried to figure out why this port problem had occurred. I wondered if women had more difficulty in the location of the port. Placement of a port above the left or right breast and under the clavicle bone apparently was common. Does wearing a bra affect the port? If you can't raise your arms above your head, how do patients pull off shirts, or dresses? Could taking off a dress or shirt over your head knock out your port? Does this mean patients can only wear button down or zipper opening clothes for eight months during chemo?

When my chemotherapy treatments continued, the process seemed to go a little better after the port adjustment. But, they were still slow and got slower each time I went for treatment.

CHAPTER EIGHT

TREATMENT SESSIONS CONTINUE

Chemotherapy #6 - June 20, 2013

At the next meeting with my oncologist, I updated her on my mediport experience and clarified just what I could and couldn't physically do. I didn't want to have another problem. So, I decided not to do my yoga or tai chi until I finished therapy. Dr. Law suggested not carrying anything too heavy or leaning over into the clothes dryer to get clothes out, and no golf swings or anything like that. I could continue my walking and could gently swing my arms. Not being able to raise my left arm also negated doing water aerobics and Qi Gong.

After I returned home from this session, more activities came to my mind. What about such daily activities using the hair dryer to dry my hair? I would have to somehow dry my hair with my right arm or be very careful not to raise my left my arm. Also, what about getting glasses or dishware down from an upper shelf or taking something out of the lower shelf of the refrigerator. All of these were most likely a no for me. I just felt the mediport catheter was becoming a real pain.

The rest of our meeting went as normal discussing what my blood test showed, and ways of dealing with side effects. Doctor congratulated me on being half way through the recovery program. She felt that considering my age (pre-baby-boomer) and all the chemo treatments, I was holding up really well. She hadn't needed to make any major reduction in the dose of chemo. My sixth stint in the chemotherapy room went a little better, but was still taking about three and one-half hours.

Chemotherapy #7 - July 11, 2013

Strange as it may seem, I began to view these chemotherapy sessions as waves in the ocean washing over me. At my seventh doctor meeting, my platelet count was found to be low, and I did not meet a national guideline for treatment. Dr. Law said that it was very common for patients to have a low platelet count at about half way through therapy because it is cumulative. Apparently every time I got a chemo treatment, the count gradually went down. My bone marrow was okay because it is able to regenerate. She started me taking B6 or B12 instead of B Complex and I would not be getting a chemo injection treatment. I was saddened on hearing this decision. I felt it was a setback in my recovery. Unanticipated tears began to roll down my face. I tried to control them and wipe them away, but they slowly continued. They were most likely my outlet for the internal pressure I was experiencing during treatment. I was given to understand that many patients cry at some point in their treatment, but it most often happens when their treatment is stopped or postponed. The doctor reassured me that I was doing extremely well, and this was normal at this stage. I said, "As long as I know that it is a normal kind of experience, I can deal with this." Dr. Law responded, "You have to remember that I am putting your body through a lot. Your body has never seen all these drugs before and you have done extremely well."

Leaving this appointment, I focused on the positive idea - I was in remission and was doing very well. As often happens in life, the delay may have happened for a reason.

A number of years earlier, my husband had a four-way bypass operation and I had nursed him during his recovery. During my months of recovery, my husband assisted me, drove me to and from treatments and was there for me during the ups and downs. Perhaps it was fortuitous that I wouldn't be experiencing the side effects of another chemo during the next week, as he was having a needed hernia operation. I would be free to care for him that week and I did.

Chemotherapy #8 - August 8, 2013

At my delayed eighth chemotherapy appointment, my platelets were still a little low, but were within the guidelines to get the chemotherapy. I met with a substitute doctor, as my oncologist was on vacation on this off therapy week for me. However, prior to this appointment, I had been in touch with her by email. I was experiencing slight pain twinges between my port and left arm. Doctor emailed me back the same day with a response. She asked if I was lifting up my left arm. I responded, "Not that I'm aware of." I had stopped Qi Gong and was trying to do more walking instead. I mentioned that the chemo nurses were still having difficulty with my port, even after the special procedure.

Chemotherapy # 9 - August 29, 2013

At appointment number nine we went through our normal routine of checking how I was doing with my side effects. Apparently my platelet count was still running a little low. I shared that once in while I was experiencing a little uncomfortable pain on the left side of the port. The nurses were unable to draw blood through the port and chemotherapy session took longer than normal. Dr. Law said it wouldn't be worthwhile to leave a nonfunctioning mediport in and would arrange to have it taken out at the end of my chemotherapy treatments.

Over the interim between chemo treatments I often felt very tired. However, I discovered that if I walked for a mile at a reasonably good pace, I actually felt better. I left our meeting feeling pretty positive, as I appeared to be on the right trajectory. My whole goal was to get through treatments so I could breathe a sigh of relief and focus on other things in my life. However, I still had to go through that day's chemotherapy. This was my ninth chemo treatment. I was three quarters of my way through the eight months of treatment. Unfortunately, this time I had my worst experience to date. The port was slow and at times shut down. Instead of taking 3-3 ½ hours, the procedure was over four hours. The nurse had to adjust and flush out the port several times. She even went to discuss the problems with my oncologist. Another port study was in order. However, I would be at a different location at the time the study was scheduled. So the study was accomplished by a different radiologist at a different hospital.

On Labor Day weekend, I woke up around 4:30 a.m. and I wrote in my journal.

I've been able to deal with reasonably good humor with all the changes, symptoms and side effects of going through chemotherapy. But this port issue is beginning to wear me down. It is hard enough to maintain a positive frame of mind when you are dealing with a life threatening illness. Although the cancer has been cut out of me, that miniscule chance that some lymph node renegades are running through my body scares me. I'm beginning to again have the feeling of concern about my life continuing. It's difficult to maintain a positive frame of mind. I need some outlet for my concerns. However, I feel and know that I'm strong enough to get through this and that we will find an answer for the port problem. Being one to move quickly to an alternative when change happens, I posed a question to Dr. Law in my email to her about the situation. Why couldn't I just get the chemo through my arm like I saw another patient receive? I do understand extensive treatments of chemo through the arm can "trash my veins", but perhaps three more times shouldn't be too bad. I'll need to check this out with her...but all this has to wait until Tuesday.

Chemotherapy # 10 - September, 19, 2013

At my next oncology meeting I was briefed on the results of the latest port study. Apparently the chemo was getting through in a "round about" way because the catheter was blocked. Dr. Law said it sounded like it took a detour through collateral vessels. I found out that when blood vessel flow is blocked, basically the body makes small vessels called collateral vessels. That's what the radiologist meant by a "round about" way. After my previous procedure, the catheter wasn't seen as blocked although it was up against the wall of the blood vessel. With the new port study, the vein was considered occluded, which means blocked. The question asked: "Was it due to a fiber like scarring tissue, or a minor blood clot? My oncologist thought she should put me on a very small dose of Coumadin blood thinner to try to keep the port open. Apparently the Coumadin medication was used as a rat poison sixty years ago. Now it was a medication? While on this blood thinner my blood would need to be checked on a weekly basis. I would have to be very careful to not cut myself accidentally as my blood would be thin and I could bleed profusely. In addition, I was concerned because I understood blood thinners weren't good in cases of high blood pressure. I had high blood pressure at one time and strokes ran in my family. Was I taking a risk with this approach?

Dr. Law thought it might take three months for the clot to open up, which did not sound encouraging to me. She felt this was the reason my chemo wasn't going directly into my vein. I asked, "How does something like this happen in this day and age?" She thought what probably happened was that the tip of my catheter, which sits next to the blood vessels, caused irritation within the blood vessel causing a clot. This felt scary to me. I've heard of people dying from clots to the brain or heart. I asked if it was dangerous and was assured it rarely travels to the heart and never travels to the brain. I was still skeptical and we went back and forth on this, because I was very worried. I didn't feel assured and pursued further questions, since I still had some serious concerns. Finally, I was told that it would be just a temporary complication and won't be a life threatening issue. My doctor said, "It's another small pebble you have to overcome." I thought at the time, if this is a pebble, what does a rock look like?

It was strange to have all these issues going on, given I'd been physically feeling better than I had felt during the whole chemo process. All my statistic assessments were good. Responding to my question as to how the chemotherapy would be done that day, the doctor said she would discuss it with the nurses. The process again utilized the port and it didn't go very well. The nurse had to flush out the port a number of times. During this time my blood was monitored, and it was decided that the small dose of Coumadin wasn't enough. The dose was increased with the addition of Lovenox injections once a day for a week. A home nursing service stopped by our home once a day, checked my stats and gave me the shot in the stomach. Not pleasant, but, I geared myself to just do whatever it takes. All I thought at the time was: I hope this does the trick and my blood meets the thinning criteria. I wrote in my journal: *I'm not sure how much more patience I have with this process.*

Chemotherapy # 11 - October 10, 2013

At my next to last chemotherapy doctor appointment I came in with a full blown sinus infection. I verified that it was okay to begin antibiotics. I checked with the doctor about how this might affect my stats given the chemo and Coumadin blood thinner treatments and received an okay. No adjustments were made to my Coumadin medication. When asked about my previous infusion, I shared the port had to be flushed several times, but somehow the nurse and I got through it. I didn't think it went any easier. Except for my neuropathy, cold aversion, balance issues, I didn't have any new side effects.

At this meeting, I believe Dr. Law prepared me for what I call "the cutting of the apron strings". She forecast I would need a full body PET scan three months after my last chemo or in January, 2014, which would fulfill my end of treatment assessment. This PET scan was important because it would be the basis on which future scans will be compared. In addition, I would need to have a follow-up colonoscopy, which was standard practice for all patients one year after surgery. I was told that, although it is extremely rare, ten percent of the cases sometimes have cancer recurrence where the bowel was connected. The colonoscopy was part of the standard of care. Also, the doctor will have another mediport study done about five weeks after I finish chemotherapy. If the study shows that the inclusion is dissolved, then I can stop taking Coumadin.

I was given the okay to go to my dentist for a checkup and cleaning. I was coming down to the wire and I, trying to keep a positive outlook, said "the mediport has been an issue, but like you said, "These things happen." This was an understatement. My Doctor suggested that it actually was a minor bump for me, and it could have been worse if I had a horrid reaction to the chemotherapy treatment. She again complimented me for making it through twelve rounds of chemotherapy. Some of the doctor's patients couldn't tolerate eight rounds of treatment and barely make it through.

She thought I was still mentally sharp, and had done extremely well. At this point I brought up the concept of some forgetfulness I was experiencing and asked about Chemo Fog. Recently, I had coffee with an old friend. She had recovered from breast cancer. My friend had asked me, "Do you experience chemo fog?" I said, "I don't think so, why?" She told me of having some memory difficulties since her cancer recovery. Once she explained what chemo fog was I had to say: "Yes, I have experienced some forgetfulness and loss of sharpness." I asked my doctor, "Does Chemo fog get better once treatment is finished?" She said, "Part of the component of the so-called chemo fog is due to the patient being so tired. We all have experienced it when we are tired and cannot focus. We have trouble remembering." Although she attempted to reassure me memory fog would not be permanent, I still felt serious concern about a number of memory lapses, and resolved to do extensive research on what is referred as "Chemo Fog" or "Chemo Brain". What I took away from this conversation is that my bone marrow would recover from the chemo treatments, but my energy level would be slower to recover. From what the doctor said that day, I thought that the longer my recuperation continued, my energy would return and the more active I would become. As the chemo worked its way out of my system; the less tired I would be. I would still be able to enjoy my life.

After my oncologist meeting, I moved on to the chemotherapy room for my input of chemo. This time when the nurse infused the mediport, I got a frightening, painful, reaction in my chest and doubled over. Several nurses rushed over to be of assistance. The infusion was immediately halted. Once the procedure was halted and the needle pulled out, I seemed to recover and shakily said: "I think I'm okay now." However, after the nurse talked with my doctor, it was decided to provide me with the chemo through a vein in my arm over the next three hours. But, my oncologist wanted to get to the bottom of why the port did not work again and what caused my sharp chest pains. So, after the infusion, she sent me right over to the hospital radiology department for (you guessed it) another port study. It showed the infusion did not go into any vein, but went into an open area in my chest. That was no great surprise to me after my negative experience that morning.

    I went home exhausted after a very long day which began at 9:00 am and ended at 5:00 pm. The next day I had an oncologist meeting planned. I also went over to the hospital for a file copy of the report and CD showing the pictures taken the day before. The port saga continued on.

    At my doctor meeting the next day, she shared a picture and explained how the port catheter was supposed to work and why mine wasn't functioning. A drawing helped me to understand just where my blockage was. Apparently, the process four months earlier was to strip away the scar band that was blocking the catheter holes. Now, the fibrous bands, plus blood product (a clot) had totally occluded (closed) the blood vessel. From what I understood, the chemo product, Xeliplatin, can be quite inflaming to the blood vessels and in my case it formed a clot.

Prior to my failed catheter chemotherapy the day before, the doctor had hoped the Coumadin, I had been taking, would have helped to dissolve the clot. Instead the nurses met resistance and I experienced pain. So, I asked: "Can't I just get my next chemo through the arm again?" I was told yes, but in order to enable the surgeon to take the mediport out, we would have to deal with the blood clot occlusion first. My doctor explained how the port is removed. If it is normally removed, more or less pulled out through an incision, this process could cause the blood clot to go to my lungs or brain. In order to dissolve the occlusion as quickly as possible, it was decided to increase the level of Coumadin and take it for two – three weeks, plus initially give me Lovenox injections daily for 7-10 days. There would also have to be on-going blood tests. I did not look forward to this regimen, but felt if suffering through it got the correct results, I could handle it. My only concern was getting my blood too thin where I could have bleeding issues. This was extensive discussion between my doctor, my husband and I about the various approaches to dealing with my problem. But, I left feeling somewhat more placated that we had an approach to deal with the latest issue and we'd see what happens.

That night I couldn't sleep well and tossed and turned. I got out of bed around 5:00 AM and excised my feelings on my computer. I wrote the following:

I'm in the middle of a health situation that I have no control over. My body is reacting to a device (a catheter) put into my body for chemotherapy infusions. Instead of working properly...it has rubbed against the inside of my vein and, over months, has developed scabbing, which clogged it up. It hasn't worked well since May (my third chemo).

Of course, it will be removed as a non-functioning port. However, the development of scar tissue (scabbing), which formed a blood clot in that area is now a serious problem. The doctors are not able to take the port out given this situation. I'm told the blood clot could go into my lungs or my brain. This scares the "hell" out of me.

Dr. Law is attempting to break up the clot by thinning my blood. For two weeks I took 2 mg of Coumadin per day. It had to be increased to 7 mg, plus daily shots into my stomach for seven days. My blood appears to have thinned to the consistency of water, based on the what I saw of the blood drawn yesterday. This regimen has really worn me down. I still attempt to take a walk or do pool exercises, but feel totally exhausted and worn out most of the day. What scares me even more, is the concern about the blood clot. I haven't been able to sleep more than an hour or two at a time during the night.

My real frustration is that I don't have any control over this situation. I'm totally at the mercy of my body and medical knowledge. I've been able to hold it together so far through this recovery process. I've attempted to be positive and utilized my inner qualities of strength, smiles, wisdom, and optimistic outlook. But, this has been a major challenge this past week. Let's hope it works out well. It's got to work out well!

Before my next meeting with my oncologist, I had picked up my port studies and had an unexpected opportunity to discuss them with the radiologist. It helped me better understand what the flow through peripheral vessels looked like. My follow-up meeting with my doctor was about ten days later when I came in for blood stats and discussed next treatment steps. The blood results affected a change in my Coumadin regimen, and they would check my blood stats again in five days. During this time frame, I also had another sinus infection and got permission to be on antibiotics – not what I would have wanted. When I asked about getting a flu shot, doctor suggested I wait until at least two weeks after I finish my last chemo treatment.

Chemotherapy #12 – October 31, 2013

Finally – it was Halloween, my last day of chemotherapy had arrived! Eight months and twelve chemo treatments later, I was done! My blood statistics were still okay for the treatment. It's hard to believe, given the ups and downs which had occurred. Dr. Law said I had done very well and got through all twelve cycles. Some patients call it quits about half way because it isn't easy given the neuropathy, mouth sores, exhaustion, nausea, etc. The doctor said, "You did it!" as she gave me a high five. She said it takes a lot of persistence and perseverance to finish the full regimen. Apparently I did well on all the measured statistics. Actually, I could hardly believe this day finally arrived. It seemed like a long term journey back in February. During the meeting we discussed contacting the surgeon for a date to remove my port. As usual, I brought the doctor up on any side effects I was still having. The aversion to cold was almost gone, but I still had to watch my diet if I wanted to avert diarrhea or constipation. I also was having balance problems when walking. She told me it related to being tired and foot neuropathy. (Discussed further in side effects chapter).

We reviewed which vitamins and supplements I should continue and which to stop. Doctor also adjusted my Coumadin dosage and regimen. Another end-of-treatment PET scan was scheduled for three months after this last chemotherapy. In closing she felt I had done very well through the therapy and didn't want me to worry about the catheter/blood issue, which was still ongoing. After January, I would be meeting with the doctor every four months for the next two years. She said now that I was finished, I had a lot to look forward to. I left saying, "I will just keep on going forward." And she responded, "Just keep going – you've got it."

After our meeting, I went into the chemotherapy room for my chemotherapy treatment and delivered homemade Halloween cookies for our nurses and other cancer patients. During the months of therapy, I would often see others graduate from therapy and provide celebratory cookies or treats for the nurses, doctors, and other patients. It truly was a Happy Halloween!

CHAPTER NINE

POST TREATMENT EXPERIENCE

Chemotherapy was completed, but post-treatment meetings continued. I went to the oncology office a week after my last chemo for blood work to monitor effects of the Coumadin, which I continued taking. I still had side effects such as dry mouth and a mouth sore. The sore was my first one while in treatment. I was experiencing a sense of total exhaustion – especially in the evenings. We were able to set up an initial appointment with the surgeon four weeks later, one and on-half months after I completed chemotherapy. I said to myself, "Finally that darn mediport will be out of my body."

Post-Treatment Meeting - November 20, 2013

Approximately a month after completion of chemotherapy, I again met with my oncologist. She was still pleased about my progress and said, "You did it with flying colors!" My husband piped up, "What about me?" and doctor said, he survived too, but I had to do all the hard work. He laughingly responded, "That's easy for you to say." It was a lighthearted conversation, nothing like when we first met. I was slowly beginning to get some energy back, but the neuropathy continued. It took six to eight months to build up the level of neuropathy and, I assumed, it would take about the same time for it to subside. It seemed my body needed to heal from all the residual side effects of chemotherapy. I received further guidance on taking a number of appropriate vitamins for a period of six-to-eight months. It was important for me to build myself up again.

I asked my doctor what else I should be cognizant of, as I moved on in my healing process. She gave me instructions on continuing to take the Coumadin. My surgeon set December 9th or three weeks from this meeting to remove the mediport. So, I would have to stop taking the blood thinner five days before this operation. Once the port was taken out, I thought I'd be home free. I asked, "How do we know that the clot will be disseminated? Do we need to take another study?" Doctor responded, "No, not before the operation because it's going to be part of the clot within the catheter." She put in a request for a Doppler Ultrasound study of my blood vessels within five to ten days after the port was taken out. In January, 2014 I was also scheduled for what is referred as the "end of treatment restaging". It is a reassessment of the colon cancer PET scan, which will serve as the basis on which my future colon assessments will be judged.

Follow-up Meeting - January 27, 2014

The purpose of this meeting was to not only follow-up how I was doing post- chemo, but to give me the results of the post-chemotherapy CAT scan and PET scan. After all I'd been through, you can imagine how relieved I was to hear my left arm and left veins were totally clean of blood clots. BIG NEWS:

Doctor declared me to be cancer free! What a joyous sound those words were to me. It was a year since I began the ordeal of my recovery journey. When asked if I had gotten back my regular energy, I had to respond "no, not quite". I did feel energetic at times, but it was short-lived and limited. I had to be careful not to extend myself too much. I needed more time and patience to recover after a year of chemo treatment. I would have to spend many additional months resting, taking care of myself and recouping my energy. I just couldn't "gun my engine and move in the fast lane" of my active life. Finally, we addressed my former ulcer problem, and it had apparently healed up, which made me think, yes, one more thing out of the way.

Near the end of the meeting, I asked about the normal process when a patient transitions back to their primary care physician. I was told usually patients reestablish their relationship with their primary care physician within two – three months after chemotherapy ends. So, after my last blood work, I would transition to my general practitioner and only meet with Dr. Law once every four months.

Side Effects - For one thing, I was still dealing with the chemo after-effects such as dry mouth, dry, crusting eyes, neuropathy, balance issues, and chemo brain. My doctor prescribed some helps, such as: eye drops, Biotiene for my dry mouth, vitamin B6 and B12 daily. I also discussed my concerns about experiencing some chemo brain issues. Dr. Law believed that my going back to my research and writing would help me keep my brain actively working. The first appointment of the new four-month follow-up rotation was May 5, 2014.

A New Start - How I felt

As this new year began, I still needed to have my after-treatment colonoscopy completed. I didn't wish to return to my previous gastroenterologist because I was uncomfortable with him and dissatisfied with the way he handled informing me of my initial diagnosis. After checking out experienced local professionals, I decided to change my gastroenterologist to one who was highly recommended. I met him in his office in January and felt comfortable with his interaction style and his experience. Thus, my follow-up clean colonoscopy was completed in February, 2014 by a new professional.

During treatment I had to postpone a number of regular check-up type of assessments. So I followed up on having a mammogram, dental checkup, and bone density assessment.

First Follow-up Oncology Meeting

I continue to have my blood taken to check iron saturation, kidney function and a cancer marker CEA. Dr. Law could tell from my body language that I felt and looked better, but apparently had some anemia based on the blood work. I may have looked so well, because I utilized the time I had to wait in the doctor's check-up room to good advantage. I completed a half-hour of Qi Gong exercises. Given how much time a patient has to wait to see most doctors, it's wise to bring along a book, magazine article, word puzzle or respond to text messages. This wait time can also be used to develop his or her list of symptoms or prepare any questions a patient might have to ask the doctor. For instance, during recovery I had difficulty falling asleep. I had tried meditation, relaxation, but these sometimes didn't work. My doctor suggested perhaps drinking some cherry juice, as cherry has natural melatonin in it. So checking possible natural ways to help you sleep may be just the key.

Update – I have continued with my life and felt it important to share my cancer journey with others, so that they may benefit from my experiences, as well as the experiences of other Cancer Survivors.

CHAPTER TEN

OTHER SURVIVOR EXPERIENCES

Each of the following persons I interviewed had a different lifestyle, background and story to tell. Yet, they all contracted the same disease and experienced similar issues on their recovery journey. I am sharing their experiences with you in the hope it will help you to be better informed as to how cancer shows itself and what one has to go through to positively survive in order to continue his or her life. Their names are fictitious, but their stories are very real.

Generally, most of the cancer survivors I spoke with didn't expect to have a cancer diagnosis. They were leading busy, productive lives. A single parent was actively involved in her vocation and raising a teenager. Another didn't know it but she was about to discover a new career. A retired gentleman was living an active sports life and traveling the world. I talked with a woman who was an avid hiker and realized she was experiencing a loss of energy and feeling drained when on long hikes. One interviewee, who had recently lost her husband after nursing him through a long, protracted illness, was also found to have cancer. I, also, interviewed a courageous, older, gentlemen in his 90's, who has survived after a stage 4 liver cancer diagnosis. I hope you find their stories assist you in better understanding the different faces of cancer.

DONNA

Donna was single by choice. She had been married several times, but preferred being single. Donna believed she was really healthy. However, her primary care doctor kept telling her at her yearly check up to have a colonoscopy. She always said no. It sounded invasive to her and since she had no symptoms, she didn't think it was necessary. Finally, when Donna was 55, her doctor convinced her to go for a colonoscopy to provide a baseline. She woke up after the procedure to find out what she thought was "seriously bad news". A tumor had grown through the wall of her rectum. It was Stage 3 cancer. She initially visited an oncologist, whom she described as very somber, with a negative demeanor. She likened him to Darth Vader from Star Wars. Donna soon changed oncologists and found one she felt comfortable with. She experienced six weeks of radiation and chemotherapy and six weeks of rest prior to having laparoscopic surgery. After a successful, but extensive, surgery she went through six months of chemotherapy and through this time mostly experienced nausea and diarrhea. She kept telling herself: "I have to keep going, I have to keep going." At the end of her chemotherapy treatments, she was extremely relieved that she didn't have to go for treatment anymore. However, she described feeling "like a wasteland inside". Through the entire recovery process, Donna maintained the attitude that death would take care of itself. If she was going to die, it wasn't that frightening. But living in a positive way had always been important to her. Thus, she decided to maintain a positive frame of mind. She had a strong spiritual base and vowed to pray and live through the treatment.

Surviving: A Colon Cancer Diary

When a friend who was a healer, suggested Donna had the talent to help others heal, she liked the idea of healing and helping people. So she decided to take a Certified Nurse Assistant course when near the end of her six months of chemotherapy. This most likely gave her a positive future reason to keep going during the difficult last weeks of "chemo" treatments. Donna said, "I completely got out of myself during the time I was learning to help others. Who knew you could get well by helping other people. It's amazing." After graduating, she obtained a job providing care in a nursing home where she could continue to help others. She believes her positive attitude and belief in God through prayer are what carried her through the treatment process. In addition, Donna had the support of her children, as well as friends, who would often show up at her house with a "big pot of soup." One hint she received from her medical advocate friend was to shut off her phone and put a sign on her door when taking a nap so she could get her much-needed rest time during recovery. When she'd meet people who asked about how she was doing, she'd answer: "I'm great, but I have cancer, can you pray for me?" She felt that her diagnosis didn't have to be a complete secret.

Donna continues to have some treatment side effects such as neuropathy in her feet, which she says actually, dulls the pain of her severe arthritis. Donna also says she continues to notice problems with balance, especially when she has to move or turn quickly, especially when taking care of her two-year-old granddaughter. In addition, she is experiencing aspects of "Chemo Brain" or "Chemo Fog" where she might search for a word when conversing. She said: "However, it surprises me sometimes when I am having a conversation and some really big words come out again. These are words that I used to use all the time." At those times, she believes she is "firing on all cylinders".

Learning's:

• Be positive and don't be afraid to have time for some solitude. During the journey, you may need time to be alone, contemplate positive outcomes and pray to God if that is your calling.

- Search out and utilize methods that can help you to deal with the side effects of chemotherapy. Donna found Reiki treatments were helpful to her. Reiki is a Japanese technique for stress reduction and relaxation. It is based on the idea that an unseen "life force energy" flows through each of us. It's said to provide healing touch energy and is administered by the laying on hands by a trained practitioner.

ROBERT

Robert had already retired from work and was living a very active sports life and traveling the world. He played golf and tennis and was doing all the things he planned to do when he retired. All of this came to an abrupt end when cancer reared its head and he had to go through treatment. He determined to go through it no matter how long it took. He said, "When you are treated, you have to take the time and do away with all the other things that you want to do. Cancer treatment was my number one priority. You have to concentrate on that no matter what." His cancer was caught at a routine colonoscopy procedure. At his age, he had never had one before, and the doctor said it was about time he got one. They found that he had stage one cancer in his colon. He said he had none of the symptoms most people have because his cancer was located in the right colon and many of the symptoms most people experienced had not occurred.

After the colonoscopy procedure, he was surprised to see his general practitioner (GP), as well as the gastroenterologist standing there. It was about four o'clock in the afternoon and his general practitioner informed him he had arranged and scheduled an operation at seven a.m. the next day. Apparently, the general practitioner, gastroenterologist and surgeon were all at the same large teaching hospital.

When asked what Robert was feeling when given this news, he said he wasn't feeling much in the way of anxiety. The whole episode was so quick – the diagnosis, the operation and the outcome, he didn't have time to think or dwell on it. He was comfortable in leaving the decisions to the doctors, because he had a heart attack fifteen years before and everything came out fine. So, because he had previously experienced a life threatening attack, he felt comfortable in going along with the doctors' diagnosis and decisions. However, the surgeon did visit him that night in the hospital to apprise him about what would happen the next morning.

Although no lymph nodes were cancerous, Robert was scheduled for chemotherapy once every two weeks for three months. His doctor selected an oncologist, and Robert felt comfortable with that because he had confidence in his general practitioner. He was administered chemotherapy through a port that was inserted in his chest by an operation. Each chemotherapy session took about five hours. When asked if he had experienced any setbacks, he said he had experienced port problems two times. The first time the port got infected; the doctor replaced the port; and treated him for infection for a couple of weeks before he could have a second port inserted. He then continued chemotherapy. Near the end of treatment, Robert's second port did not operate correctly due to fibrin clot, and he ended up receiving chemo through the vein in his arm. Unfortunately for Robert, near the end of his therapy, the infusion of chemotherapy drug, Oxaliplatin caused inflammation of the vein that leads to temporary arm swelling. In spite of all his problems, Robert strongly believes in getting chemotherapy treatment. He could not say enough about the nurses in the oncology center. He felt the attentiveness and kindness of well-trained oncology nurses helped get him through the physical and psychological part of his cancer journey and recovery.

One of the side effects or results Robert experienced after going through chemotherapy treatment was an increase in cavities in his teeth when he had his next dental visit.

Robert contracted cancer three times over a period of ten years. Each was caught early and did not spread. He firmly believes in catching cancer early. When something is wrong, check it out. He said to a doctor once: "Can't we watch it and see if it doesn't grow more serious?" The doctor said no.

Surviving: A Colon Cancer Diary

Learning's:

- Robert learned it is a mistake to not check health issues immediately because if you wait, it will grow to be more serious because the cancer can develop and spread. He says, "Bite the bullet rather than waiting to see how it goes. Deal with it and move on."

PAULA

Prior to her cancer diagnosis, Paula was working and led an energetic, busy life throughout her sixty-two years. She's an avid hiker and lives in an area with mountains and trails. One day, while hiking, she realized that she'd been gradually losing energy. Her hikes were becoming more and more draining on her. Next, she noticed blood in her stool when she went to the bathroom. Her general practitioner thought it was probably hemorrhoids and said not to worry. However, Paula insisted on having a colonoscopy because she had an older sister die of cancer.

The colonoscopy resulted in locating three tumors, one of which had broken through the colon wall. Paula was devastated and wondered how this could have happened because she had been so vigilant due to her family's cancer history. Over the last twelve years she had colonoscopies done every two or three years. The doctor always found a large number of polyps which were snipped and taken out.

Paula had to wait a month after diagnosis before surgery could be performed. For Paula and her husband, it was the longest month of their lives while they waited and comforted each other. They finally met with the laparoscopic surgeon and he operated to remove the tumors. The surgery was successful, but one tumor had broken through the colon wall and affected lymph nodes. This meant that Paula had Stage III cancer.

She was then referred to a local desert oncologist, who explained the surgery results and suggested a treatment plan of chemotherapy with a Mediport. Meanwhile, Paula did research on the Internet of various treatment options, but after a while decided to stop torturing herself looking at the various methods of curing cancer. She decided to just buy into the chemo program, which gave her an extra 20% protection of killing renegade cells. She wanted her life back. She encountered one problem in having a port. Initially, when she was doing floor pushup exercises, she opened the insertion wound; the port moved out of place and had to be adjusted by the surgeon in a second operation.

Paula believes dealing with chemotherapy is different for each individual. She says she has a personality where she wants to have all her ducks in a row. She wants to be in control of her life. However, when Paula would drive a long distance for chemo treatments and find she has to reschedule chemotherapy due to inadequate blood counts for treatment, she found it frustrating and depressing. This made her realize she no longer had control. She thought, the sooner I come to grips with that fact, the easier time I will have with this process. She said, "Initially, I wanted to control my appointments, my treatments, and my body." When Paula did have her chemo treatment, she would allow three what she called "down days" where she had no expectations, no energy, and could rest and recover. She was then back taking her long walks or hikes. To walk or hike was not only a way to help Paula work out any chemo side effects, but also helped to increase her energy level. Often exercise helps a person increase his or her energy level. She hated taking medicines for nausea and took them only when absolutely necessary.

Initially when Paula began her cancer journey, she and her husband waited to tell family members and friends until they had exact information. From then the family was updated on her condition and progress by emails, phone call and Skype. When friends would call she would say "I'm doing fine. I'm going on a hike."

Initially, when Paula's diagnosis was verified, she called her younger sister to inform her. She found her sister had not had a colonoscopy for three years. Paula encouraged her to get another procedure right away, since she was diagnosed and their older sister had died of cancer at 47 years old. The family may have what's referred to as Lynch Syndrome*. Her sister also tested positive for Lynch Syndrome and was found to have a cancerous tumor. So both she and her sister "walked the same cancer recovery path" for eight months. They supported each other and talked frequently during the months of treatment. Paula said it was helpful for each of them to share the ups and downs of their cancer journey.

Paula had twelve treatments and always kept a count of the number of times she had left. However, you can't count on a schedule exactly because there are times your blood work or white cells might not meet the criteria and your chemotherapy might be postponed. This is always a disappointment because once you gear yourself for the next treatment and are turned away, you either feel sad or relieved that you won't have it that day.

Paula experienced several chemo side effects. One was a serious sensitivity to anything cold, especially cold drinks or cold air for a few days after each infusion with one of the chemotherapy drug, Oxaliplatin. When she was outside in the cold air or drank a cold drink, her throat appeared to close up. She solved this problem by buying and wearing what are called Survivor Buffs. She would wrap her neck, mouth and head in the buffs to keep warm when she walked in the early morning. When walking or hiking, she also wore running gloves to keep her fingers warm and wool socks to warm her feet. At home she'd drink liquids at warm or room temperature. In addition, Paula had a severe case of neuropathy in the bottoms of her feet. She said it felt like walking on a sandy beach twenty-four hours a day with grinding sand between her toes. She solved this by wearing socks at home. Three years later, she still wears socks in the home. She has some lingering side effects in her feet which feel tingly, but says this is slowly coming around and the throat issue is resolved. Although her sister lost her hair during chemotherapy, Paula's hair thinned, but she never lost her hair. She attributed her hair thinning to taking Biotin hair supplements during treatment. She was prescribed medications for treatment of chemotherapy associated neuropathy.

She has experienced one side effect referred to as Chemo Brain or Chemo Fog, which affects quick recall of names, or other information in conversation. However, what has helped Paula is to be back at work greeting cancer patients who come in for treatments. Helping them and relating to them is something she feels good about. She now feels 100 percent normal and has learned not to dwell on things. Paula understands that patients aren't considered cancer free until after five years, but she felt cancer free the moment she had her last treatment.

Learning's:

• An important learning for Paula and others is that knowing family history of cancer is vital, and if a person finds or knows of cancer in other members of one's family, it is extremely important to get genetically tested for a condition called Lynch Syndrome. Because Paula's sister had defective repair genes, she and her sister have had their families tested and screened with colonoscopies and tests for Lynch Syndrome.

• Prior to her cancer journey, Paula believed she had control of things. She knew exactly what she was doing and where she was going in her life and in her home. She was in complete charge of her life, her home, the cooking, the finances, and the household. During therapy, she had to let go of these responsibilities and found her husband of 37 years picked up the slack and did amazingly well.

- Some of the changes Paula has experienced is she has a greater appreciation of life. The flowers are brighter. Little things are more important. She has a need to spend more time with people she cares about. She realizes that life is finite and it's more important not to waste time. She's learned to take action on and do the things she wants to do and not wait or put them off. For both Paula and her husband, it's acting on their retirement plan and "bucket list".

JOAN

Joan's life had dramatically changed in the period prior to receiving her cancer diagnosis. Her second husband had died from a protracted illness – liver cancer. She was in her sixties and had been his caretaker for a number of years. When growing up, she had developed caretaker skills by caring for her younger siblings and was comfortable with the "Mom" role. After her husband died, she said she went into a "funk" or deep depression for about one and one-half years. This is when she began to experience erratic bouts of diarrhea as well as an uncomfortable, unwell feeling in her abdomen. Her doctor put her on antibiotics, thinking she had an infection. The doctor didn't ask her when her last colonoscopy was. Four months later, she went back to her doctor again and said: "This is awful. I can't live like this. I'm living on Imodium." Joan asked about having a colonoscopy. The doctor checked her file and didn't have a colon report on file and sent her to a gastroenterologist. The doctor asked her when she had her last colonoscopy. It turned out that Joan had a colonoscopy eight years before done by a doctor in another state, where she had a second residence. That's why there was no record in her primary care doctor's file. Initially Joan had an endoscopy done because she has a history of ulcers. That test was negative for ulcers. Next step was a colonoscopy. After the procedure, the doctor kindly and with care told her she had cancer. Her reaction was "so what's our next step?"

Her thinking at the time was that she would die of cancer and be with her husband, her mom and dad, or she would live and be with her grandchildren. She didn't care if she lived or died.

She next went with her daughter to meet with an oncologist who carefully explained what would need to be done with surgery and chemotherapy treatment. Chemotherapy was begun six weeks after her successful surgery, when Joan recouped her strength. Joan spent seven hours per session for several months receiving chemotherapy. Treatment began with infusions every three weeks. When Joan got treatments, she talked with people around her because they were all in the same boat. She said it might seem strange to people in the general public, but chemo time was for many patients a time to socialize with others who understood what they were going through. There was a sense of camaraderie since they were all going through therapy. She would often read her book, then talk to people and go back to her book.

She refused help from friends and family who were willing to drive her to and from sessions. She drove herself. Joan felt she needed to be strong and not be an "invalid". She was invited to lunch by friends and initially said yes, but later cancelled. On days after chemotherapy, when she felt really sick, she didn't want to bother getting dressed up and going out to lunch. Initially, Joan felt she didn't need help and shopped for her own groceries loading up on food and water the day before her chemo sessions. Her daughter scolded her for being so stubborn and independent. Her daughter said: "You don't have to be the strongest woman on earth. You are hindering getting better by pushing yourself."

After a few months into the chemotherapy, Joan developed a reaction to the chemo that scared her. She felt terribly ill and ended up sleeping on the bathroom floor for three hours. After this, she decided to stop "being totally stupid" and began to accept help. Looking back, she realizes her family and friends were just trying to be part of her getting better and recovering.

Joan's daughter gave her own email to Joan's friends so that if they couldn't reach Joan one day, they would call her daughter. But there were days she didn't feel like talking or was too sick to answer the phone, so they would call her daughter. This upset Joan, and she berated them for doing this. But, later regretted doing that. Now, she believes you have to be honest and explain to friends some of what you are going through in treatment.

The major chemo symptoms Joan experienced were weakness and nausea. The nausea was treated with pills. The weakness was represented by an exhausted feeling. She took care of herself and rested when she felt tired, weak and lethargic with no energy on the first couple of days after her chemotherapy session. She would just sit in a chair and watch television. When she felt better, she would get up, get out of the house and go in her car for gas or groceries. Other symptoms Joan experienced were headaches, a red face, red eyes and red hands. She said she probably looked like an alcoholic without a red nose. She is also experiencing what she calls brain muddle. She has had minor episodes of forgetting something, which may be what's referred to as "brain fog."

Now that her chemotherapy treatments are finished, she plans to celebrate. She said, "Now I don't have to account to anybody. I can finally make plans without asking permission."

Learning's:

- One of the things Joan learned is that chemotherapy takes its toll on the human body. In therapy you are given a lot of toxins, which not only kill bad cells, but some good cells as well. You don't know what it's killing other than cancer.
- She also learned to be more open to asking and receiving help from her family and friends. She realizes she didn't need to go through the difficult days of recovering alone. She learned that if you move to a new location, be sure to access your medical records or get them forwarded to your new physician.

ALAN

Alan was no stranger to cancer. His mother had rectal cancer. After a colostomy operation, she had to wear a bag, as he put it. His older brother died of stomach cancer and his youngest brother died of Hodgkin's Lymphoma. Thus, Alan, who is 95 years old, was not surprised when he was told he had cancer by his oncologist. A mass in his rectum was cancerous and had metastasized to his liver. He was diagnosed with Stage 4 cancer.

Alan's health history included a heart attack over ten years before and surgery to place a stent in his heart. He said he woke up after that surgery and things were great, thanks to the surgeon who saved his life.

On his most recent health emergency, he had bleeding from his rectum and drove himself to the hospital emergency and was then admitted to the hospital.

His cancer treatment consisted of initial radiation treatment to stop the bleeding from the rectal tumor and then intravenous chemotherapy infusions consisted of Avastin and chemotherapy. Alan did not have a port inserted in his chest because his chemotherapy drugs are not the type that would irritate his veins. He received his chemo infusions through his arm. His only problem was that his blood was thin due to taking aspirin, and this caused him to have black and blue marks where the needle was inserted. He took aspirin because of his heart vessel stent and to prevent blood clot from one of his cancer treatment drugs, Avastin. Alan took combination of Avastin and chemotherapy until the total disappearance of cancer in his liver. He now receives maintenance treatment with Avastin to prevent cancer recurrence. When asked if he has had any difficulties or hit any treatment roadblocks, he said the worst part was when he saw the insurance statement as to the cost of receiving the necessary drug.

Alan's daughter and family live approximately 150 miles from him. He's quite independent person and lives alone. He has limited support from a neighborhood program and has someone check in with him each day. He's considering getting information about contacting a medical alert or personal emergency alert company, someone he could call for help in an emergency. Recently, he tripped over an extension cord in his garage and experienced a bad fall. Luckily, he was finally able to get up, didn't break any bones and just scrapped his elbow.

Alan's recent CAT scan showed no evidence of any cancer. His view of cancer is that it was there and it's being treated. When he might feel depressed, he gets to thinking positively when he goes for therapy and sees people who are much worse off than he. He also enjoys talking with and getting a hug from his favorite nurse at the chemotherapy center. He appreciates the positive attitude of the nurses who staff the chemo room.

Alan says "Thank God for the computer." He plays solitaire, watches news on Yahoo or on his television and keeps up with world events. Once in a while he drives the 150 miles across Los Angeles to Malibu where his daughter lives. His sage advice for someone beginning cancer treatment is to "keep a positive attitude as things could be worse."

SANDRA

When cancer interrupted Sandra's life, she was a single mom, working and raising a teenage son. She led an extremely busy life, yet carved out time for volunteering and friendships. Her cancer diagnosis definitely forced her to put her life on pause. She said the most challenging thing when she was first diagnosed with colon cancer, was figuring out how she could adjust her busy life.

It started when Sandra felt a very sharp pain on her left side underneath her rib cage in the middle of the night. She assumed it was some kind of digestive issue. The pain went on for ten hours before it dissipated. Over the next weeks and months, the pinching pain would sporadically occur, but Sandra didn't think it was anything serious – probably just related to what she was eating. Since she thought she was really healthy, she'd not been to see any kind of doctor in eight or ten years. In February, Sandra went to see a gynecologist for a check-up, PAP smear, breast exam and blood work. Although her blood work didn't show anything unusual, the gynecologist suggested she monitor when she experienced the pains and obtain a checkup with a general practitioner. As she became more aware of the pains, they seemed to come more frequently. Friends told her the pain was a sign that something was wrong, and they insisted she go see a doctor. So she did. After reviewing her CAT scan, the doctor asked her if anyone in her family had colon issues. She said, "Yes, I had a brother who at 46 was diagnosed with stage 4 colon cancer." After finding out she had not had a colonoscopy, he scheduled her for one. The colonoscopy showed she had a tumor which was soon operated on. Unfortunately, the tumor had broken through the colon wall infecting one lymph node of twenty-four collected. Sandra had stage three cancer.

She had sailed through the surgery and felt it wasn't a "big deal" for her. Sandra thought it would take several weeks to recover from the surgery, and she felt she could continue work and her activities through the period she would receive chemotherapy. Sandra wanted to be a fighter and didn't want to let down others or make more work for other people. It didn't take long for her to realize she had to take care of herself and put herself first to get through the months of therapy.

After recovering from surgery, Sandra selected several people who she felt could best assist her through the difficult months of chemotherapy. First, she chose an oncologist she could relate to and who was a right match for her own personality. Next, she selected a friend/counselor she could meet with to discuss her feelings, issues and ways of maintaining a positive mindset throughout therapy. Then she picked someone who could help her to eat healthy and chose appropriate foods. Finally, Sandra selected a personal trainer who would work with her to develop a regimen of exercises which would assist her to stay strong and physically able as she went through months of therapy. By obtaining assistance from the medical field, nutritionist, exercise trainer, counselor and her Christian church spiritual supporters, she felt she had the best approach to survive this overwhelmingly difficult time in her life. As Sandra began therapy, she initially thought she should eat a healthy diet of fruits, vegetables, salads, berries, Kale, Kiowa, etc. However, during chemotherapy, she experienced such severe stomach cramps when eating these foods, she realized that what is good for you when you are well, is not necessarily what you should eat during chemotherapy. Her oncologist suggested she eat such foods as crackers, rice, eggs, bread, and pasta, which would be easier on her digestive tract. Now that she has completed the chemotherapy regimen, she is gradually introducing "healthy foods" back into her daily diet. The major complaint Sandra had during treatment was her difficulty in having to take too many pills each day - vitamin supplements, medication, etc. Her son said that was the only time she ever complained.

Sandra spent four to six hours getting intravenous infusion of chemotherapy drugs at the oncology center. She would wear a small machine which dispensed the chemo for the next forty-six hours, after which she'd have seven days off. Approximately at round seven, of the twelve total rounds prescribed, Sandra felt so sick, she broke down and cried at the thought of having to go the next day for treatment. She required a treatment break for her treatment side effects during her treatment course. Although she fought to have a great attitude towards treatment, due to her body's reaction, she had some difficult days.

However, when she received a delay, the tension she carried in her body receded and she felt better. After a difficult bout with side effects, Sandra came up with an idea to gear herself up the day before her next treatment. She requested her friends and family send her "crazy fight songs" as a motivation. She was deluged with such songs as; the music from the movie, *"Rocky", "I Will Survive"*, and *"Shake It Off"* by Taylor Swift, Christian hymns, etc. These helped her to cope with the anticipated therapy expected the next day. Christian hymns were important to her because they were soft, soothing and comforting when she felt her worst. They reminded her of what is good in the world.

Sandra utilized Facebook to inform people of her diagnosis and asked that they pray for her. Because Sandra is involved in her Christian Church and has been of help to others, they were there for her. They supported her in a variety of ways through her treatment and recovery. Many friends volunteered, and it was up to Sandra to determine how best to utilize their skills. When she felt her worst during chemotherapy, family and close friends were there to care for her. Other friends did her grocery shopping, cleaned her house, and even walked her dog when necessary. Two friends always went with her for her doctor's appointments. One drove, while the other went in to the doctor's office with her and took notes. That allowed her to listen to what the doctor said, without trying to take notes too. People encouraged her throughout her treatment on Facebook and through texts, emails, calling and in person.

Sandra believes the number one resource in going through recovery is a patient's attitude. She confirmed this with her oncologist and her counselor. How a patient perceives the illness can either help or hinder him or her to heal. One has to fight to live, fight to have a great attitude. It was more important to her than the treatment she was given or the foods she ate.

Although Sandra continued to be active and do some of her activities on the "good" days of this recovery journey; after chemotherapy was completed, she was able to go right back into her work life, without "skipping a beat".

Learning's:

• By experiencing and living through her recovery process, Sandra said she gained a deeper level of compassion for people who are sick and suffer through a long term illness. She realized the importance of adjusting her regular diet due to the effect of chemotherapy on her digestive system. She noticed the importance of keeping a regular exercise regimen to keep her strong and maintain stamina and circulation of her body on chemotherapy treatment.

- We can all learn the importance of not only reaching out to friends and family, but finding concrete ways to utilize their offers of help. Sandra made lists of all the people who wanted to help her and put them into categories of what she felt comfortable in letting them help her do. Whether it was taking her to the doctor, doing grocery shopping, cleaning her house or making a casserole for supper, she had to learn to utilize their skills.
- Songs and music can be a positive way to raise one's spirits. Sandra believes singing songs for ten minutes a day can actually make your left brain and right brain work together. Because going through therapy can be stressful, singing happy songs can help change a person's mood and the way he or she is thinking. She said: "A person can't help smiling when they sing "Zip a Dee Do Da, Zip a Dee A, plenty of sunshine coming my way...."

PENNY

Penny was a pilot and has flown most of her adult life. Prior to her colon cancer diagnosis, she hadn't been getting colonoscopies. She was apparently losing weight and thought it was a good thing since she had wanted to lose pounds. One day she was watching television, while exercising on a treadmill and heard Katie Curic talk about her husband's colon cancer which caused his death. Penny was noting the signs of colon cancer – one, two three, four, five and she was saying, yes, yes, yes, yes. Yet, she said, "It can't happen to me." She now admits that she was in total denial.

She was experiencing constipation and didn't think it was unusual. However, it got a lot worse and this continued for about a year. To deal with it, she was taking laxatives, but at some point they weren't helping anymore. So, she finally went to see her family internist about the problem. He set up an appointment with a gastroenterologist since she was bleeding a little. He performed a sigmoidoscopy and told her he couldn't see anything. He thought it was probably fissures. Penny returned to her primary care doctor and reported on the findings, but she felt there was still a problem.

Her primary care doctor arranged for a barium enema and X-rays, which showed there was a problem. She was able to obtain a prompt colonoscopy due to the seriousness observed by her physician. The colonoscopy showed the blockage and a biopsy was taken. She had a stroke of luck, in that a surgeon was able to fit her in the end of that week. Although this was her first major surgery, she said she didn't have time to be scared for long. At the time it felt scary, but she also adopted a mindset set-that, she would be okay. Her primary care doctor was present for the surgery and told her that they took out 38 lymph nodes, and he assured her everything was okay. Reflecting on the experience, Penny said she was mentally upset at the news, but things progressed so quickly, she didn't have time to be scared. Also, she had emotional support from her mother and a dear friend, which helped her to pull through it. Before this experience, Penny had never had a colonoscopy. She was fortunate that the surgery was successful in ridding her of the cancer and no cancer was found in her lymph nodes.

Learning's:

- She did not have to experience chemotherapy and feels she was very fortunate. She now has a colonoscopy every five years.

CHAPTER ELEVEN

MANAGING CHEMOTHERAPY SIDE EFFECTS

Opting for chemotherapy, which is a systemic treatment to kill cancer cells located anywhere in your body, means that you will be also killing rapidly dividing healthy cells. Patients going through chemotherapy experience a variety of side effects such as dry skin, rashes, mouth sores, depression, hair loss, fatigue. The side effects a person experiences, depends on both the kind of chemotherapy he or she is being given and their body's' ability to deal with the chemicals.

Before you begin chemotherapy, your doctor will provide you with all the facts about treatment, including the drugs you will be given and the side effects you may experience. You may experience none of them or a few different ones. Generally, most effects gradually go away after treatment ends and healthy cells grow normally. However long it takes to get over side effects will depend upon the kind of chemotherapy you are given and your overall health.

    HAIR LOSS - One of the side effects that are most familiar when people hear someone is on chemotherapy is hair loss. Hair loss generally begins 2 or 3 weeks after the chemo treatment begins. How much hair loss involved also depends on the type and combination or regimen of chemo drugs being given a patient. In my case, my friends and family were surprised to see that I still had my own hair, although unbeknownst to them, it did thin out a little. Patients, like a neighbor of mine, who do lose their hair, often shave their heads shortly after beginning treatments and get a fashionable wig to wear until their hair grows out. The good news is that hair does begin to grow back typically 1 – 2 months after chemotherapy ends. In my own experience, it isn't growing as thick and quickly as before my chemo stint.

DECREASED APPETITE - Often patients tend to lose weight when they've been diagnosed with cancer. In treatment, one of the issues is decreased appetite sometimes due to anxiety or depression. Also, the chemo drugs may cause food to taste different – more sour, or bland, or there may be a metallic taste in the mouth. However, it is important to maintain your weight and your strength through treatment. Often nutritional supplements and vitamins are prescribed. I was lucky enough to have a friend lend me *Eating Well Through Cancer,* which had all kinds of recipes not only for nutrition, but the book; was broken down into sections. If I was dealing with diarrhea or constipation etc., there were recipes which would help me to deal with those issues. I would encourage readers to check on line for cookbooks and nutrition books recommended for their type of cancer recovery.

DIARRHEA - Your gastrointestinal GI tract cells can be damaged by chemotherapy causing diarrhea. If diarrhea continues it leads to weakness and dehydration and needs to be controlled. It's important to notify your doctor if the diarrhea doesn't clear up in 24 hours, or if you have a fever, severe cramps, or bloody stools. People who have had surgery on their GI tract, tell me they've experienced a change in their bowel patterns. They sometimes have to go to the bathroom six-to-eight times per day and even during the night which interfered with their rest and sleep.

NAUSEA AND VOMITING - Although less common and less severe, some patients experience feeling sick to their stomach. Often your doctor can prescribe medicine to help. It helps to breathe deeply and slowly when feeling nauseated. Distraction also helps to take your attention from feeling sick. Some distractions which can help are chatting with friends or family, listening to music, watching TV shows or a movie. Other helpful hints are to eat small mini-meals throughout the day, rather than three big meals. Eating and drinking slowly also help to control that sick feeling. You might have cooked cereal such as Cream of Wheat or oatmeal for breakfast. Snack on crackers or pretzels. Other easier foods to digest are pasta, white boiled potatoes and baked or broiled chicken. The important thing is to chew your food well. If strong cooking smells bother you, try to eat foods at room temperature or cold foods. Another trick when you feel nauseated is to breathe deeply and slowly. Utilizing meditation can also be helpful.

NEUROPATHY – Certain chemo drugs can cause neuropathy, especially when higher doses or after multiple doses are administered. Peripheral Neuropathy may be acute or light during or shortly after continued cancer treatments. What happens is one or several of your peripheral nerves have difficulty sensing information. It often affects a patient's extremities – hands, fingers, or feet leading to weakness, imbalance or numbness. Neuropathy can last a few days in some instances, or can be chronic and recur over a period of time after treatment. How it may feel is a tingling or pins and needles or numbness in your fingers and toes, especially as a response to cold. Neuropathy can be triggered by eating, drinking or touching something cold, or even breathing in cold air. Depending upon how much a patient is affected, he or she may have difficulty buttoning a shirt or picking up small objects. Neuropathy in the feet can cause problems with balance or walking. My experience consisted of having a light case of neuropathy in my fingers and feet. I would have to really concentrate on keeping my head erect looking straight ahead. If I turned my head right or left looking around while walking, I tended to weave to and fro like how a drunk might walk. Often patient's neuropathy symptoms may improve or resolve within six or twelve months. But for others, the symptoms may last for a longer period of time. For other survivors it may become permanent and this may restrict their daily activities.

PAIN – The chemo drugs can damage nerves leading to numbness, tingling or shooting pain – often in the fingers and toes. Some drugs can damage nerves to the extent that a patient experiences shooting pain often in his or her fingers and toes. Other drugs can cause mouth sores, headaches, muscle pains and stomach pains. However, not everyone with cancer and receiving chemotherapy experiences pain from the disease or the treatment. If a patient is experiencing pain, he or she should immediately talk with their oncologist. Be prepared to tell your doctor where you feel the pain, what it feels like – sharp, dull, throbbing, steady? How long does it last? What eases the pain or what seems to make it worse? You most likely will be asked on a scale of 1-5 to grade your level pain. Pain may be managed with medicines, relaxation, exercises to lessen tension and reduce anxiety.

CHEMO BRAIN OR CHEMO FOG --- This is a term which describes thinking and memory problems cancer survivors experience after cancer treatment. Cancer survivors have worried about or joked about what is termed chemo fog or chemo brain. Its exact cause is yet unknown, yet many survivors can attest it is real. Most survivors, including myself, find it somewhat frustrating when searching for the simplest words, ways to express themselves or when forgetting the name of a friend or acquaintance. To combat this, what survivors do is try to work their brains by doing crossword puzzles, SUDUKO, Word Jumble, writing memoirs, reading and taking notes on what they read. However, even with these antidotes, there are still times I have to search my mind for a name, let's say of a movie actor or even a friend, and berate myself for not knowing. But, most survivors have learned to accept that chemo fog is real. When a person forgets, he or she may concentrate for a while, and often the name does finally surface. If the name doesn't come up, just fess up and ask the person his or her name and move on.

CHAPTER TWELVE

SUPPORT SYSTEMS - FINANCIAL, FAMILY, FRIENDS

FINANCIAL

When cancer strikes, what you don't need is to worry about who will cover the expenses. You need to focus all your energies on fighting the disease. That is why it is important to obtain and maintain health insurance – personal or public. The Affordable Care Act (ACA) provides easy to read guidelines about cancer coverage and how the ACA helps cancer patients and their families.

It may be strange to say, but I was fortunate to have contracted cancer, when I was retired and had Medicare Insurance plus good personal healthcare insurance. It relieved me of money worries, so I could focus on what I needed to do to fight the disease. This is why I was thankful that I maintained a good healthcare policy over the years. I didn't have the additional worry about paying the entire treatment bill.

FAMILY AND FRIENDS

When a person is diagnosed with cancer, everyone around the patient – spouse, partner, relatives, children, grandchildren and friends are also impacted in some way. The diagnosis might come as a surprise, and they might feel paralyzed as to what to do. They may not know what they can do to support the cancer patient. Initially, the patient may not know because he or she is wrestling with the prognosis, recommended operation and/treatment. Often assistance and help depends on the circumstances and nearness of a supportive family and/or friends, as well as the needs of the cancer patient. Visiting them in the hospital, offering to do shopping errands, making foods that they like and are able to eat, driving them to oncologist appointments and chemotherapy sessions are a few ways someone can help. Why not send fun greeting cards and/or notes to the recovering patient while he or she maneuvers through recovery? Keep in touch occasionally online or with text messages. Let them know they are being thought of and wished well.

When you contract cancer, how you handle it is a very personal decision. Some people are more private than others. While some cancer patients may go online to send out emails or blog about their experiences. Others tend to pull back to be alone or retreat into their family circle. Some cancer patients immediately join a cancer support group, while others prefer to do their own research and information gathering. There is no one right way for everyone. However, what interviewees have shared with me and what I experienced is on-going support, which I found to be beneficial to my recovery. Being in touch with others can help you expand your knowledge of what to expect, how to treat side effects, and provide nurturing when you have a "down day".

I personally took a middle-of-the-road approach. I maintained what I called "get well" time where I did the activities I felt well enough to do, but tried not to over extend myself. This was usually in the morning or early hours of the day. What I found is activities had to often be impromptu if I felt well enough at the time. Planning events way ahead during chemotherapy can be an "iffy" situation, because you may have to back out because of not feeling well enough to go.

I believe the approach I chose was the most plausible for me. I kept my immediate family updated by phone, emails and in person when possible, since they live some distance from us. In order to reach other friends in our community, as well as distant family members, I occasionally sent out an update about my condition and progress. I often received well-wishes and responses which I would answer. The advantage of utilizing emails, rather than receiving phone calls, is that you can interact on the computer when you are feeling your best. When experiencing a difficult day, you don't necessarily want to see or talk with anyone. After beginning chemotherapy, there are days you just focus on recovering, "vegging", watching TV or reading. You find ways to take your mind off of your condition.

Surviving: A Colon Cancer Diary

As I began exercising and taking long walks around my extended neighborhood, I met new people I'd never met before. They'd engage me in short conversations, and I learned a lot about nutrition and cancer recovery.

Exercise was one of the keys to recovery per my doctor, so I would set up what I called "walk/talks" with various friends. It's amazing how fast the time goes and the distance you cover when walking and talking. An additional benefit was that I could keep up on friends and activities in my community, despite initially not attending various events. When I couldn't walk outside, I walked on an indoor track with my husband. I didn't rejoin my water aerobics class because they did arm reaching exercises which I felt may jeopardized the port lodged in the upper left portion of my chest. So I developed my own water aerobics routine which stayed within my capability.

During the day, I worked at the computer writing my memoirs. My cancer scare woke me up to the importance of leaving behind a personal history and legacy for my family. Prior to experiencing cancer, I had felt healthy and thought I had a lot of time to work on memoirs. So, my first priority was gaining back my heath. My second prority was writing my memoir stories for my family. I would write early in the day, but by early evening I felt tired and exhausted. I would sit or lie on the couch and read books or watch TV shows or Netflix.

Gradually, I began to interact more with friends by attending various activities in our retirement community, such as my book club, music concerts, and a few dinner events. In my experience while in chemotherapy, I felt the worst shortly after therapy. Much of what a recovering patient can do depends on his or her side effects and how they affect their life. I was able to write at the computer most days; presented several scheduled conference seminars on my first book, *Changing Lanes,* and fulfilled a number of speaking engagements and book signings. The rest of the time, I concentrated on resting and getting well again.

Other cancer patients I interviewed had their individual ways of dealing with family and friends during their recovery process. Some reached out to family and friends utilizing their help and assistance. Others preferred to personally deal with cancer treatment on their own or within their family and pulled into their protective shell. However, those who did reach out found that friends were ready, willing and able to provide a "big pot of soup" or do an errand or provide a ride. Often family members and friends don't know what to do for you or what you might need. They shy away because they don't want to bother you during recovery. But it's important to reach out not only to the patient, but to the family as well. Keep in touch and find out what is needed – offer your help. I did recently telephone an ill friend. Both she and her husband were down with the flu. She took me up on my offer of help and asked me to go to the store for groceries they needed. If you are the patient in this situation, don't be afraid to ask for help. One interviewee utilized the services of a personal trainer to help her exercise, a nutritionist for an appropriate diet and spiritual counseling from her church connections. They helped her to successfully recover, and I'm sure they felt rewarded in the process of helping a friend in need.

Another support system which individuals who are diagnosed with cancer can seek out for help is the *American Cancer Society*. Their website is:

www.americancancersociety.com.

Another source for connection and information is a *Gilda's Club*. Clubs are located in various communities, so check to see if there is one in your area. This organization provides professional programs of emotional and social support, education and fitness for everyone or anyone affected by cancer. They assist patients going through treatment, caregivers, family, loved ones, children and those managing chronic cancer. The club is also a haven for cancer survivors and people who have lost a loved one to cancer.

CHAPTER THIRTEEN

FINAL THOUGHTS AND SUMMATION

When going through cancer treatment it's essential to maintain a positive attitude because, when you think you have one problem under control, often another one arises. If you view these issues negatively, you'll begin to feel overburdened or downtrodden and won't be able to deal with them effectively. A successful recovery demonstrates how important it is to have a positive attitude and open mind about the various prescriptions to unexpected medical problems which arise in one's cancer journey. This can sometimes be easier said than done. Maintaining that positive attitude can be extremely challenging at times. I know from experience. I had to struggle with a non-functioning port after being told such problems were few and far between. Whenever

I faced issues that could go wrong though rare and, few and far between, I had to disregard negativity and keep my mind focused on winning my cancer battle. I survived four rounds of chemo through a problem functioning port and succeeded in getting the twelve rounds of chemo regimen – the last one through a vein in my arm.

In the end, I wondered if my cancer journey might have been easier if I had been more knowledgeable about cancer and more familiar with others cancer experiences. That's why I have shared my experience and interviewed other cancer survivors as to their personal experiences. Although this is primarily a book about one personal experience, it encompasses the knowledge and expertise of medical professionals, as well as other patients, who have successfully gone through their own survival journeys. One of the precepts in cancer survival that I've learned is: when you think you have one problem under control, often another issue arises. If you view each of these negatively, you won't be able to deal with them effectively. You just have to take them on one at a time. The personal stories in this book demonstrate how important it is to have a positive attitude and open mind about various prescriptions to unexpected medical problems which arise during one's cancer journey.

The goal in sharing the stories and information in this book is to help those who are diagnosed with cancer to have a productive experience and recovery. The journeys others have traveled and what they learned may help others to experience their own successful recovery. Each chapter includes "Learning's" from those of us who have successfully survived, as well as explanations of terms in the Addendum. These can save you time in researching definitions and meanings. However, I do encourage you to go on-line and research cancer treatment and survival ideas, as there are new advances being made in the field.

Beverly A. Battaglia, Ph.D

EXPLANATION OF TERMS

GLOSSARY OF TERMS USED IN THIS BOOK

ADJUVENT THERAPY – is additional treatment used to increase the effectiveness of primary therapy. It may follow after surgery to increase the possibility of curing the cancer or prolonging remission. Adjuvent therapy may consist of chemotherapy, radiation therapy, biologic or hormonal therapy

BONE SCAN searches for the spread of cancer in your bones. It is also used to evaluate arthritis, healing bone, or infection. A radioisotope injection is given, which is taken up by areas of the bone where cancer, inflammation, or injury is located. A camera is used to locate and record anything that looks suspicious. Abnormal areas light up the scan.

The injection is usually out of your system within 6 – 24 hours.

CT/CAT SCAN (computerized axial tomography) is actually an x-ray showing organs and tissues as three-dimensional, cross-sectioned images. The patient has to lie still on a table which moves through a doughnut shaped machine which takes pictures of various parts of his/her body. Sometimes a dye containing iodine is injected first so specific blood vessels and other tissues are clear on the image. New spiral CTs operate faster and provide more detailed pictures.

MAMMOGRAPHY is a low dose x-ray machine that provides a detailed image of the inside of your breast and identifies any abnormal areas, such as tumors and cysts. Two or three images are taken from different angles to get a complete image of the whole breast area.

MRI SCAN (magnetic resonance imaging) is a scan which creates three-dimensional, cross-sectioned images of a patient's tissues and organs. As a magnet transmits radio waves through the body, the images get projected onto a computer screen and film. An MRI requires about 30 to 60 minutes.

PET SCAN (position emission tomography) is a scan of your whole body looking for abnormal sugar consumption increases, which can be a sign of cancer cell growth. The results are correlated with other abnormalities seen on other tests – i.e. CT scans. A PET scan is utilized to diagnose early cancer, detect the spread of cancer, and monitor cancer treatment response.

ULTRASOUND utilizes high-frequency sound waves and their echoes to make images of your tissues and organs. When sound waves hit something solid, their echoes are bounced back. The rest of the waves go farther until they hit a solid area. Thus, a two-dimensional, black and white picture is recorded on a screen. A gel applied to the patient's skin in the area of the ultrasound, improves the transmission of sound waves and their echoes. New ultrasound technology not only shows more details by creating three-dimensional images, but also analyzes several two-dimensional images which can help in early detection and treatment

>Reference Source: *Diagnosis & Treatment – Tests Use During Cancer Treatment"*

Caring4Cancer, Winter, 2013

Beverly A. Battaglia, Ph.D

ABOUT THE AUTHORS

Beverly Battaglia, Ph.D. is a retired social psychologist, consultant and university instructor. In her consulting practice, she assisted clients deal with the aspects of change, in order to be successful and productive. Now retired, she utilizes her change expertise to help others adjust to the twists and turns of change in retirement. Her book, ***Changing Lanes: Couples Redefining Retirement*** aids couples in successfully dealing with the changes experienced transitioning to and in retirement.

Beverly is a colon cancer survivor and this book describes how she and other cancer survivors overcame obstacles in their recovery journey. Beverly lives in Southern California with her husband, Steve. They continue to lead busy, active lives in retirement and share a love of travel.

Amy Law, M.D. is the medical consultant who contributed to this book. She is a Diplomat of the American Board of Internal Medicine and Medical Oncology. She is a partner at Desert Hematology - Oncology Medical Group, Inc. in Rancho Mirage, California. Dr. Law played a major role in Beverly's recovery and was instrumental in providing information and guidance for this book.